WAITING

for the

MONSOON

Rod Nordland

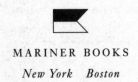

MARINER BOOKS

New York   Boston

To Fredney

Pages 249–250 serve as an extension of the copyright page.

HarperCollins books may be purchased for educational, business, or sales promotional use. For information, please email the Special Markets Department at SPsales@harpercollins.com.

FIRST EDITION

Designed by Renata DiBiase

Library of Congress Cataloging-in-Publication Data has been applied for.

ISBN 978-0-06-309622-6

23 24 25 26 27 LBC 5 4 3 2 1

And did you get what
you wanted from this life, even so?
I did.
And what did you want?
To call myself beloved, to feel myself
beloved on the earth.

RAYMOND CARVER, "Late Fragment,"
from *A New Path to the Waterfall,* his final book
of poetry, written as he was dying of lung cancer

Contents

Contents

PROLOGUE

My Second Life

The following article was written from my bed in the Weill Cornell Medical Center's neurology ICU and published on a full page of the Sunday edition of the *New York Times*.

"WAITING FOR THE MONSOON"
By Rod Nordland
New York Times, September 1, 2019

I routinely give titles to my journals, in which I have long recorded interviews, appointments, odd thoughts, and cris de coeur. My journal commencing June 17, 2019, is called "Waiting for the Monsoon."

The Indian summer has always fascinated me, and I was in New Delhi, experiencing its climatic extremes firsthand.

Summer is when the heat of the subcontinent's vast plains generates an enormous mass of warm air that pushes against the impenetrable massif of the Himalayas to the north, while the west wind drives clouds from the broiling Arabian Sea across the country.

Heat builds to inhuman levels: days of 125 degrees Fahrenheit are not unheard-of; 110-degree days, or 43 Celsius, are common, with humidity sometimes approaching 100 percent.

These are the forces that breed the southwest monsoon, the greatest accumulation of fresh water in the atmosphere anywhere on the planet, and it broods over a landmass with the earth's densest population: 1.3 billion people. The poorest of that multitude suffer grievously from heat and thirst, but all are waiting for the monsoon to bring relief.

For weeks in June and July, black clouds gather as the entire country obsessively tracks the progress of the rains.

The waiting is a time of expectation and worry: if it rains 10 percent more than normal, it means catastrophic flooding; 10 percent less may mean drought and famine.

The high drama of the wait was captured by the fifth-century Indian poet Kalidasa:

> *The clouds advance like rutting elephants,*
> *Enormous and full of rain.*
> *They come forward as kings among tumultuous armies;*
> *Their flags are the lightning; the thunder is their drum.*

Then one day comes "the bursting": all that fresh water breaks as if from a celestial womb, gushing as much as 40 inches in a few weeks.

When the universal longing is finally requited, there is a sense of nationwide relief, bringing with it an almost immediate respite from the terrible heat. Temperatures drop overnight by an astonishing 20 to 30 degrees.

On the morning of July 4, I left Delhi for Uttar Pradesh to report a story on India's feverish toilet-building campaign. I was out on the street most of the day when I noticed ink in my journal was smudged with raindrops. "The monsoon has arrived," I noted.

The smudged page also contained a fragment of overheard conversation: "We will marry our daughter to you only if you have a foot." It was the first line of an intriguing story I would never write . . .

The next day I went for a morning jog in Delhi's beautiful Lodhi Gardens. [It was 120 degrees Fahrenheit at 10 a.m.]

That is really the last thing I remember with certainty. I only learned later that I had . . . made my way from the gardens to New Delhi's Golf Course Colony, several miles away.

This is where a malignant brain tumor, as yet undiagnosed, struck me down and left me thrashing on the ground.

A Good Samaritan, I would be told, had seen me reeling in circles, with arms upraised, as if dancing, or praying, then watched me collapse in an epileptic seizure [which doctors later said had probably been a grand mal seizure, judging from the extensive bruising on my body].

He hailed an ambulance, which sounds strange . . . although in India, one hails an ambulance like a taxi, a practice sometimes abused by wealthier citizens . . . to avoid epic traffic jams. The ambulance drivers would not, at first, take me to a hospital unless this Samaritan—Sunny Kumar Kangotra, an aid worker at a private foundation—came with them.

They were concerned about being blamed by the police for a thrashed-up foreigner, and they wanted Sunny to take responsibility for me.

But doing so meant he would have had to leave behind his motorcycle, one of the two most valuable things he owned. After a lot of haggling, he offered to follow behind the ambulance, but the crew worried he would race off.

So Sunny negotiated a compromise: he would give them his

second-most-valuable possession, his smartphone, as a guarantee that he would stay with them until they got to the hospital. Since the phone meant a month's salary to him, he did not give it up lightly.

The driver for the *New York Times* bureau in Delhi, Jagmohan Singh, had already realized something was wrong when I had not returned within the hour I had promised. Jag, as we all called him, has worked for multiple bureau chiefs over the past 20 years and he remains friends with many of them. He began doggedly ringing the cell phone I had in my pocket until finally someone answered it and told him I was on my way to Moolchand Hospital.

We foreign correspondents depend heavily on our local staff members; they are our interpreters to their societies, our protectors, our surrogate families, and they often become great friends as well. But I was new to Delhi, filling in for our bureau chief, Jeffrey Gettleman, while he was on vacation, so the bureau staff barely knew me.

Nevertheless, as I heard later, half a dozen of them gathered with Jag around my hospital bed, sending an important message in a country where your place in a byzantine social hierarchy can be a matter of life or death. It was, in short, a crucial communication: that this is someone to attend to.

Now the monsoon was upon us with a vengeance. Reflections of lightning flashed across the walls of the intensive care unit, and sheets of nearly horizontal rain beat a tattoo against the windows, with seemingly no spaces between the raindrops.

While I was comatose for a day or two, dozens of people perished from the flooding in Mumbai in early July.

My journal picks up again on July 8, a Monday, with the pages of the preceding weekend blank, as if they had disappeared from my life. I noted the absence with dismay.

At that point, I had been moved to a private hospital, and my journal was full of puzzlement about what had happened. After my run, a seizure, but what was that even? At first I posited heat stroke from exercising in extreme weather.

Dr. Rajshekhar Reddy, the head of neurology at the Max Hospital, was in charge of my case. He told me what I had, but only in the most circumspect manner.

"A sub-cranial, space-occupying lesion," he said.

"A what?" My skepticism of that euphemism shouted from the page.

Then, for reasons obscure to me, the following pages are devoted to collective nouns for groups of beasts.

A cauldron of bats (what else, Lord Macbeth?).

An obstinacy of buffalo (of course).

A cackle of hyenas (ha ha).

A conspiracy of lemurs (hee hee).

A crash of rhinoceroses (indeed).

And one I already knew: a murder of crows (kaw kaw).

A prickle of porcupines. I had no idea where I acquired these terms, perhaps from a talkative and literary-minded nurse.

Clearly, I thought, this was my mind showing off, saying, "Hey, I'm still in here, regardless of any alleged 'space-occupying lesion.'"

I found that term annoying: it sounded like a pointless euphemism for a tumor, and I said so to Dr. Reddy, who smiled enigmatically but kindly. "We cannot call it a tumor until we can biopsy it and we find tumor cells."

All I could do at that point was laugh. The whole experience was becoming increasingly amusing. I frequently laughed out loud, however bizarre that might have seemed under the circumstances.

I was still seizing up, or so witnesses would report. The

medical team would have to induce a coma to get the seizures under control, and at one point (this is hearsay, but too good not to recount), I was taken for dead by a mortuary crew, who toe-tagged me with the following ID: "Unknown Caucasian male, age 47 and a half."

Nothing could have cheered me up more. It was only days until my 70th birthday. "Well," I thought, "I could learn to love this tumor."

The age-flattering toe-tag was, it would turn out, the first of several silver linings caused by the stunning impact of this cerebral intruder in my life. They say that people who survive malignancy of this magnitude approach it with a positive attitude, and I was determined to be one of them, not a victim swept along by bad weather and worse luck.

The next day, I was medevacked by the *Times* from India to New York–Presbyterian Hospital's Weill Cornell Medical Center, one of the best hospitals in America.

Back in India, the monsoon was in full swing, once again, as from time immemorial . . .

The rains were inundating the fields of the farmers who have to feed a billion mouths. Those brown fields were green again, and the floods devastated some areas.

The sheets of rain would eventually drain off into the Arabian Sea, whence they came, or into the Andaman Sea to the east, to which they had been bound.

As for the ebbing of the space-occupying intruder in my head, that remained to be seen. From 3 to 6 percent of glioblastoma patients are cured; one of them will bear my name. I've already ordered a T-shirt with a giant 6 and a percent sign on it.

The monsoon lasts all summer, so it is raining in India as I write this. In the meantime, I am teaching myself to love my tumor. Hopefully, love it to death (its, not mine). It has not just made me younger by about 23 years, in toe-tag time, but it has made me better, somehow stronger, funnier, even kinder, more tolerant. Ask anyone who has seen me lately.

I think of my tumor cells as a hawks' boil—the collective noun for two or three raptors when they circle their prey. And when my oncologists come around to discuss the progress of this disease, to them I assign a collective noun that I had underlined, thrice, presciently, in my journal: "a shrewdness of apes."

In the Weill Cornell shrewdness troop, Dr. Phil Stieg is an alpha male, chairman of neurology and neurosurgeon-in-chief. He was my brain surgeon and there was from him no politely indirect talk of space-occupying lesions. His bluntness came as a refreshing breeze. "It's a glioblastoma multiforme," he declared, naming the worst, most aggressive of brain tumors, "and I'm taking it out right away."

He sawed right in and resected what he said was 99.99 percent of it from my brain's right parietal lobe. The remaining 0.01 percent will be radiated and treated with chemotherapy just in case.

"We're on a journey," he said.

Dr. Stieg has a podcast, the title of which I have borrowed for my current journal, which opens on my 70th birthday, which was also the day Dr. Stieg operated: "This Is Your Brain."

I'm done with waiting for the monsoon.

"I need to talk to you," Dr. Stieg said as I crouched on the toilet in my ICU room. When I asked if he could wait a minute while I finished, he told me what he had to say couldn't wait, and he kept talking.

"This disease will kill you and you need to come to terms with that.

"Tell your children, tell your family, they need to know the truth. Your median life expectancy from diagnosis is fifteen months. We can maybe buy you some more time with good treatment, and we will of course try to do that. This is a journey and we're just starting on it, and I'll be with you the whole way; but understand that it will get you. It's a terminal disease, it's incurable, and it will eventually kill you."

It will eventually kill you . . .

Dr. Stieg's crisp verdict arrived following my brain surgery, during which he extracted a lime-sized mass from my right parietal lobe. I was recovering in the intensive care unit, where I would stay for a week. After that, I spent the next three weeks moving into different hospital units, all geared toward making me whole again, or at least as whole as I would ever be with glioblastoma now a defining part of my physiology, if not my identity. My next stop would be the neurology ward and then off to the rehab unit for intensive physical, occupational, and speech therapy. The hospital was like a massive educational facility from which I would matriculate with all the skills necessary to beat the odds against a disease that most people die from in fewer than eighteen months.

But at least I had company. My partner, Leila Segal, had accompanied me every kilometer from Delhi, on the long and perilous (for me, as I was riddled with embolisms) flight to New York. Leila is a poet and a writer and human rights activist, who already had an Indian visa from our earlier trip there together and flew there as soon as she was notified of my hospitalization. She arrived just a day later, in time to help my nurses restrain me from getting out of bed. She has barely left my side since then, dealing with doctors, with my employer, with mind-numbing logistics, not to mention with me, the man she had planned to make a life with, who now wasn't always present or functional, much less the person she had fallen in love with.

July 17, the day of the brain surgery to remove my tumor, also happened to be my seventieth birthday, and all of my loved ones had gathered in my room beforehand. Close friends, like my fellow *New York Times* foreign correspondent Alissa Rubin and my decades-long friend Matthew Naythons, MD, a physician and a photojournalist; also, my five siblings and some of their spouses and even children from Philadelphia. Most astonishing and most heartening was the presence of my ex-wife, Sheila, and my three children with her. I had been estranged from them following my separation and then divorce from their mother. There they all were. My second daughter, Johanna, a professional photographer and capoeira instructor, then living in Spain; my son, Jake, who was on his way to graduating magna cum laude with a bachelor's degree in foreign policy from the University of Sussex; and my eldest child and first daughter, Lorine, who was working in Britain on a master's degree in sustainable development.

But this was a highly curated group—even my telephone calls were blocked unless the caller knew the password, "Batman," after the nickname a long-ago girlfriend had given me. They were all very protective of me, gatekeepers wary of my volatile temper and careful to weed out and block visits from people I thought of as ghouls, sort-of-friends who just wanted to see what a man marked for death actually looked like. I felt protected and cared for and, above all, beloved, but I was also intensely aware that gathered around me were my freshly-ex-wife and my new partner (who, slightly to my horror, I saw settled together in a corner for an hour-long tête-à-tête along with my eldest child, Lorine, whom everyone agreed was the one most like me). In my absence Lorine was de facto running our family, if only by the sheer force of her personality and bristling intelligence. Not all these people liked one another, but they were all there for me, and I hoped would remain there for me in the hard months and years ahead. I felt bathed in their collective presence, this assembly of love and caring. I reflected then that in all my life I had never been so happy.

"It will eventually kill you . . ."

It's not as if death, specifically premature death, was alien to me. After all, before I became an international correspondent-at-large for the *Times*, I was the chief foreign correspondent for *Newsweek* and earlier the Asia correspondent for the *Philadelphia Inquirer*. For nearly five decades I had faced down death, my own or others', covering virtually every war of note from Cambodia in 1978 and on through East Timor, Sudan, Bosnia, Somalia, Chechnya, Kosovo, Iraq, Yemen, and finally Afghanistan. In total, I reported from 150 different countries—ten of them in 2018 alone, the year before my disabling tumor struck. Most of these states—Nicaragua, Afghanistan, Iraq, Lebanon, Syria, Congo, Yemen, Bosnia—were going through violent upheavals; I ran war-zone news bureaus in six of them. There was the guerrilla in Cambodia, with a bullet in his head, convulsing in the back seat of my rental car. His distraught, heavily armed comrades insisted we get him to a hospital immediately, "or else!"—even with half of his cranium and a lot of his brains splattered over the Avis upholstery. Getting him to a hospital, where he was destined for the morgue anyway, meant illegally crossing an international border and risking imprisonment by some aggressively unpleasant Thai soldiers. But, just as in that intensive care unit at the Weill Cornell Medical Center, I never had any doubt I would survive.

In 1979, working on an article about ruby smugglers in the Karen State of Burma, an area better known as the Golden Triangle, the source of much of the world's opium and heroin as well as smuggled gemstones, the rebel commander of the Shan State Army was hosting me and Matthew Naythons, then my photographer, in his command post when heavy gunfire woke us all up. As Burmese government forces began to overrun the immediate area around our bunker, he offered us these words: "Don't worry, guys, we'll never let them take you alive."

"That's OK," Matthew coolly interjected. "Let them take us alive, please."

In 1979, I was reporting on factional infighting on the Thai-Cambodian border, at the Khao-i-Dang refugee camp (then the biggest in the world), when I acquired what for years was a prized possession: the Shirt of a Thousand Holes. At a border checkpoint a group of militiamen had demanded the key to the trunk of my car, which I pretended not to have. So, with a light machine gun they rock-and-rolled on the trunk, which held only suitcases of clothing, now riddled with bullet holes. One once-nice white shirt, short-sleeved, was especially badly shot up. Later I took it to a tailor and asked him to sew up every hole, whereupon he came to the conclusion that the Shirt of a Thousand Holes had only three hundred holes, which was very decent of him, since I was paying by the hole. I wore it proudly for years.

So yes, death was no stranger to me, and yet, when Dr. Stieg delivered this blunt news, as much as I appreciated the honesty, I couldn't assimilate it as easily as I had my on-the-job near-death experiences. I suppose I was truly shocked because the news immediately set off a seizure.

I struggled to face the immense implications of what was happening to me. It was all disorienting and terrifying. My tumor stripped away my autonomy, my sense of the future, and certainly a few cherished aspects of my identity. And I will get to those losses. But something else happened that was even more profound: only a few days after my collapse in New Delhi, I embarked on my Second Life, an experience that I can only describe as one of the greatest gifts I have ever received.

The famous French neuroscientist David Servan-Schreiber is

one of many philosophers of cancer who talk about the phenomenon of the Second Life; faced with a terminal diagnosis, most people realize that they really have two lives, and the Second Life has
just opened up to them. It is a life of doctors and impairment and
uncertainty, to be sure, but also of some surprising beauties and
benefits. One of them being that a terminal diagnosis makes them
appreciate even more their First Life. That, at least in part, is why
so many of them talk about how much of an improvement their
cancer has made in their lives, their new lives, their Second Lives.

Inevitably, my long absences, and the traumatic nature of my
work, undermined my marriage and family life. Lorine, a child of
the Bosnian conflict, was born in 1992; Johanna, a child of the Iraq
War, in 1995; and Jake, a child of the war in Afghanistan, in 1998.
I didn't appreciate until much later how my constant travel to war
zones affected my children—all the missed birthdays and family
events and personal milestones of my children. I was instead proud
of myself for never mistreating my wife or any woman or child, as
my father had done to those around him.

In my mind, I had made astonishing efforts to go home as frequently as I could, even while covering wars that were front and
center on the news agendas of the organizations I worked for. From
the early 1990s, I ran a *Newsweek* bureau in Sarajevo. My family
was living in Italy, and I commuted there for weekends, via a French
C130 Hercules cargo plane sponsored by NATO on behalf of the
UN Protective Force. I flew from Sarajevo to Ancona, where I had
stashed a car—an old but very fast secondhand BMW M series—
drove the two hundred miles to Rome on Friday nights, and came
back to Sarajevo on Sunday nights. It had to be one of the world's
strangest commutes. My journey began like this: from my seventh-
floor room in the Holiday Inn Hotel, a building often shelled by
Serb forces on the opposite mountainside, I would don my hel-
met and body armor—which in those days weighed a good thirty

pounds, with breast- and ballistic backplates of carbon-steel alloy. I'd use the stairs down to the basement because elevators were far more dangerous when shells hit the building. Then I would get into the armored car I shared with the *Washington Post* staff, drive up the underground garage's exit ramp, and at the top make a high-speed turn out of the building, knowing that snipers zeroed in on that exit. I'd drive over the curb of the adjoining road and across a grassy verge, keeping the vehicle's trajectory as unpredictable as possible, then swing onto Zmaja od Bosne Boulevard, better known as Sniper Alley, for good reason. I'd hear bullets pinging off the car's armor and hope they weren't the .50 caliber projectiles of Russian sniper rifles, which could have pierced that armor like butter. Once at the airport, I would board the NATO transport, a C130 piloted by French air force officers. I would sit up front with them, which I appreciated, because the cockpit seats had five-point seat-belt harnesses instead of the flimsy lap belts on the fold-down canvas jump seats in the cargo hold.

I tried to do the same sort of commute from Afghanistan, and later from Iraq, where just the act of getting to the Baghdad airport was heart-in-mouth scary on the most dangerous mile of roadway in the world at the time, dubbed "Route Irish" by the military. We tried relocating the family to Beirut, hoping I could commute there on weekends. It was a road trip lasting ten to twelve hours, which seemed doable—but alas, that road went through Fallujah, soon to be in Al Qaeda's hands. In 2005, I told Sheila *Newsweek* was promoting me to the post of chief foreign correspondent (my dream job), and she told me she wanted to separate, which we did.

But here we all were, crowded around my bed in the cramped hospital room, among wires and monitors, and tubes and IVs bristling from my arms, the machine showing all my vitals beeping away. I amused everyone with a trick I had learned; by staring at the monitor showing my pulse rate, I could will my pulse down, just by thinking about the number on the screen; and as I breathed deeply, it would drop to the number I was mentally commanding it to. I had arrived at the hospital with a resting heart rate of fifty beats per minute, normal for me; doctors at one point asked if I were a marathon runner and seemed skeptical when I denied that. At one point, I alarmed everyone by pushing my RHR down first to forty, then thirty-five, which triggered alarms and prompted Jo to cry out, "Stop it, Dad," as she had in so many other situations. When I looked at the faces of my children, and those of my dearest friends and loved ones gathered at my bedside, I knew, perhaps for the first time, how deeply I was loved. If a fatal brain tumor was the price I had to pay for that, I considered it a fair bargain. The assembly of all my loved ones in my ICU room, as they all got the grim prognosis, was reassuring and affirming, and I think it marked the official beginning of my seventh decade and my Second Life. There were complicated family dynamics at play (what family has no complicated dynamics?). Clearly, this gathering could have gone haywire in many ways—with so many family members and friends, my ex-wife and my new partner, how could there not be difficult emotional crosscurrents? And yet, something profound had happened, we were all in this together, and we would continue to be. I reflected then, not for the only time during my hospitalizations, that I had never in my life been so happy.

This is hard for people to believe or understand, but glioblastoma multiforme stage 4 has proved to be the best thing that ever happened to me—maybe even if I don't survive it, but especially if I do. I have come to think of my tumor as my friend, my teacher, my mentor, and especially, my *gift*.

The profession of medicine, like journalism, is inured to black humor. Thus, some doctors have nicknamed GBM-4 "The Terminator" because of its resoundingly aggressive nature. About 250,000 cases worldwide appear annually, and it's the disease that very publicly killed Senators Ted Kennedy and John McCain and President Joe Biden's son Beau. Among malignant primary brain tumors, it is probably the most common and the most aggressive and deadly. As far as I was concerned, I was going to make the best of it. "The brain tumor was long overdue," I wrote in my journal shortly after the surgery. "I'm going to overcome this and suck it for all it's worth. We should all be proud of ourselves." I resolved to become the best brain-tumor patient in the world. Six percent of us with GBM-4 do manage to survive five years without recurrence, and there was no reason why I could not be in that elite group.

In the months that passed after my stint in the hospital, I was fully inhabiting my Second Life. I no longer flinched at love and intimacy but exulted in its balm and power. In my Second Life, my children and I made peace and enjoyed a closeness I had once thought impossible. In my Second Life I could see clearly, finally, all the mistakes I had made in my first one. Gone was the old arrogance, the certitude that dominated my every action—a combination that likely helped make me a successful foreign correspondent and bureau chief but denied me the opportunity of becoming so much more.

Friends and family members and editors have often raised their eyebrows at my frequent assertions that my tumor was the best thing that ever happened to me, a gift that has enriched my life ever since. They are skeptical about my full embrace of this Second Life. But I know that I am not alone in this experience

"Disease, age, and life itself prepare us for death," Rabbi Steve Leder wrote in his marvelous book *The Beauty of What Remains*. "There is a time for everything, and when it is our time to die, death is as natural a thing as life itself." The Buddhist monk Frank Ostaseski, who for many years ran the Zen Hospice Project in San Francisco—which provided end-of-life care for the homeless and AIDS victims—put it another way: "None of us get out of this alive." He has sat with thousands of some of society's most marginalized people on their final journey. "Not one of them were afraid," he wrote in his book, *The Five Invitations*.

Several months after my brain tumor and I were introduced, I decided, unprompted, to reconcile with an old, long-ago lost friend from Philadelphia. Larry Moskowitz and I hadn't spoken in twenty years, after a close personal friendship of twenty years. Many times, mutual friends had tried to persuade me to reconcile with him, and I had just spurned all such efforts. This time I just realized it was the right thing to do and approached Larry, who reached right back. We had known one another almost half a century—what a waste those silent years were for us both. Once we began talking, it was like we were picking up a conversation that had begun decades ago and had never really stopped. We tried to remember exactly what ridiculous spat had driven us apart, and we both realized that whatever it had been, we had long ago forgotten it. We both agreed that each of us had been assholes. (Privately I mostly blamed myself and thought Larry was just being generous, as usual.) As Larry left my apartment he said, "I love you, buddy," and I said, "Same here, old friend." Now I regard him as another brother, and wish that we could do as the ancient Romans did and adopt new siblings.

"None of us are making history when we die," Rabbi Leder said, "and in many ways, all our deaths are the same." Yes, I understand that now too, and I find it oddly comforting.

My diagnosis brought a little extra laughter to my life. It even made me better in mundane ways: I have stopped drinking, and I have lost fifty pounds, partly because of abstaining from alcohol and partly due to strict adherence to the keto diet of high protein and fat, with almost no carbs. It has been proven scientifically to be effective in killing cancer cells, and for the first time since age eighteen, I am back to my fighting weight—literally. I was for a brief time a semi-pro boxer in North Philadelphia, a paid sparring partner but not a prizefighter in the light heavyweight class, at 165 pounds. I now brush my teeth three times a day. I never did that but once a day, or even a week if in the field. A small thing? Not if you're my teeth.

The day my "Waiting for the Monsoon" essay ran in the *Times*, David Remnick, the editor of *The New Yorker*, wrote a note of congratulations. In it he called me "the foreign correspondent's foreign correspondent." I treasure this even more because Remnick is, himself, a consummate foreign correspondent. "You have always been," he wrote, "one of those reporters whom everyone who knows anything looks up to. And your essay today . . . will outlast the lot of us."

My reply to David explained something about why I do what I do (though I should now say "did," since I will not soon be flying off again to Afghanistan, my most recent foreign stomping grounds). "One of the great things about being a foreign correspondent," I wrote, "is that the material is often just so damn strong. It's what has kept me at it so long. In what other job, for instance, are you going to get to explain the heart-wrenching dynamics of a family where all seven sons had their limbs blown off by a piece of accidentally triggered ordnance? Such stories are nearly always inspirational looks at the human condition. The wounded boys lay on stretchers outside at the hospital on a fine day, with their schoolbooks hidden under their pillows—they were desperate to study for upcoming national exams and afraid the docs would try to stop them to make them rest. It's hard to write about, on one hand, but it is hard *not* to write about. One instinctively 'storifies,' as you editors say. That is even more true of one's own catastrophic illness; and if I couldn't make something compelling of it, I wouldn't be much of a writer."

That essay became the inspiration for this book, and is reprinted in the opening pages. Before my illness people would often say, to my slight embarrassment, "You lead such an adventurous life," to which my reply was always "The only true adventures are adventures of the mind."

GBM is a physically and mentally disabling disease. There was no longer any possibility that I would be that roving war correspondent, going to places no one else could get into all over the world.

Writing this book, while enduring the often harsh treatments for brain cancer, became my adventure of the mind. Writing it restored my freedom, dignity, and sense of self-worth.

My Second Life has certainly made for some compelling material. But my First Life is what got me here, and that's where this story begins. As Confucius is reputed to have said, it is only when confronted with your second life that you realize you only really have one life and finally appreciate it fully. Here goes.

PART I

Before the Monsoon

"UNDER INDONESIA, TIMOR
REMAINS A LAND OF MISERY"
Philadelphia Inquirer
May 28, 1982

DILI, East Timor . . .

Bernardo, 56, who lives with his wife and 10-year-old son, sat on the bare dirt floor of his house, which was devoid of possessions of any kind; there was also no sign of food in the house. Asked how the harvest had been, he surveyed the circle of officials and, after a long pause, said, "There is not enough to eat."

The next house was identical, except that nine persons lived in it and that it contained a piece of furniture, a table. Under the table—the coolest place at midday in the tin house—lay a boy sweating and shaking in what his family said was a three-day-old malarial fever. Other children in the household had bloated bellies and emaciated limbs. Thomas Ferreria, the family spokesman, was asked through an interpreter about his family's condition.

"Tell him," Maj. Marsidik warned Ferreria in Indonesian, "that it's OK here."

Ferreria did as he was told.

"So even though the crops are bad, you have enough food for the whole family?" he was asked, in English.

"Tell him you have enough until the next rainy season," said Marsidik in Indonesian.

"We have enough until the next rainy season," Ferreria said.

CHAPTER 1

We Called Her Mommy

I was the oldest in a family of six, with a preternaturally abusive father, Ronald James Nordland, and an astonishingly patient and saintly mother, Lorine Elizabeth Myers.

My mother's childhood was the stuff of so many Depression stories; she was buffeted by wild swings from prosperity to penury. She would describe going to the beach at Ocean City, New Jersey, as a little girl, in a private railway car, one of the privileges of being the granddaughter of a wealthy real-estate developer in the Philadelphia area. And then, her father invested heavily in real estate in North Philadelphia just as the phenomenon of white flight to the suburbs turned that part of the city into a slum; he was bankrupted before moving to the suburbs himself. Before that happened, she was the only white girl in her North Philly high school.

My parents met immediately after World War II, when my father was a dashing sailor fresh off a tour of the Pacific with the US Navy, on a destroyer that berthed in the South Philadelphia naval yards. She was an exceedingly impressionable, quite beautiful seventeen-year-old and was swept off her feet. My father was blond and handsome, born in Norway and brought to the States when he was a baby. His family moved to the West Coast, and when he and my mother eloped, she dropped out of her Philly high school at age seventeen and they moved to California. Where he insisted they have a big family, for reasons that would only become apparent years later.

Whatever remained of that whirlwind romance was soon eclipsed by the beatings, the violence in our home, the exhausting pregnancies, and many hastily forced moves, but this chapter is about my mother—how she protected us and how, in the words of the Christian hymns, she was our rock and our salvation. My father's story merits its own chapter, which follows.

Our early childhood years were spent in rented houses in various Southern California communities—Rialto, Riverside, San Bernardino, Colton—but the one I remember the best is Fontana, a far suburb of Los Angeles in semi-rural San Bernardino County. The town is best known as the birthplace of the Hells Angels motorcycle gang. As a youngster I remember watching, agape, with all the other neighborhood kids, as they cruised, reclining almost all the way back on their choppers, two or three abreast, driving around the circular and figure-eight lanes of our community of ranch and split-level single-family homes—arrogant in their scruffy leathers, with their "colors," denim jackets with the Hells Angels insignia, on their backs. Like most people in the area, our family kept animals in the backyard—mostly chickens and turkeys. We raised and ate them. My father was very efficient at slaughtering them, and we would sometimes see turkeys running headless around our yard, blood spurting from their necks. I didn't find it especially traumatic, except we did sometimes have issues with the chickens because, as children do, we would name them and make pets of them, imploring our father not to make us eat "Polly." Or whomever. The turkeys, such disagreeable creatures, were much less likely to be treated as pets.

The back of our yard abutted the desert, with a tall row of eucalyptus trees demarcating the property line and providing perches for the chicken hawks that occasionally preyed on our poultry. When I first went to kindergarten, I had to walk by myself a mile through the desert to get to school. My father showed me the route and how to manage it, a memory that is uncontaminated by darkness or danger—just a dad looking out for his son. We never lived in any of our many California homes (ranch-style or split-level houses, usually with a carport) more than one school year, often less. My mother later worked out that we moved an average of once every six months—common in those days, especially in California.

It's funny, but the few good memories I have of my father during my childhood in the 1950s—trout fishing in the High Sierra, firing off CO_2-cartridge-propelled balsa wood rockets in our front yard—somehow seem to be in black and white, like nearly all TVs in those days. But my memories of the terrible beatings he so often committed are more in Technicolor, which also arrived in the 50s, at first only in movie theaters. Even as a young boy, I came to realize that my father was some sort of criminal—there was the sudden middle-of-the-night scurry to empty the house of our belongings and stuff them into a trailer kept in the carport, the move to a new house in a new town—but I didn't know what kind.

He worked as a mechanic in a service station, so I imagined him to be some sort of car thief.

Once the family of a female first cousin on my father's side came to visit us for a weekend. The girl and I spent happy hours playing house together in our carport, using cardboard boxes to build our playhouse; I would have been between six and nine years old then, she I think about the same, so I'm sure our play was pretty chaste. Those were some of the happiest hours I remember from my childhood, but they ended abruptly when her parents suddenly dragged her from the carport, got into their car with her, and left. For months afterward, I asked my parents when my cousin might visit again, but my inquiries were met with an embarrassed silence.

My mother was an incredibly forgiving soul: she blamed her-self—as so many women do—for her husband's angry abuse. When I was much older, in one of our late-night talks she confided that when my first sister, Cynthia, was born, she was suspicious of my father and took care to keep him away from their daughter, which she said deeply wounded him and explained his angry abuse. That had been unfair of her, she said, because she was quite sure that he had never abused any of his own children sexually.

Her suspicions were hardly unfounded. If I had been older at the time of my cousin's foreshortened visit, I might have worked out for myself what had happened. My father was no car thief. He was a predatory pedophile and had probably tried to abuse my cousin, his niece. Much later in life I learned, to my horror, that he was repeatedly arrested and often convicted of sexual assaults on children, both boys and girls.

Apparently, he favored physical violence when he attacked us. I repeatedly lied to concerned school authorities about things at home because I knew even then that telling the truth would inev-itably lead to a very bad place, one involving the police and arrest warrants and probably vengeance attacks, or even state-compelled foster care.

From the time when I was very little, my mother shared almost everything with me—we were both night owls by nature and typi-cally she would talk to me after midnight while doing the ironing or some other housework. I don't think she had any close friends then. At least no friends close enough to address her by her nickname, Mickey, as her sister and parents did from childhood on—and as my father did during the good times. In one of those wee-small-hours-of-the-night conversations, when my father might have been out of town or trying to evade authorities, she warned me that even in the 1950s, in semi-rural Southern California and hyper-conservative San Bernardino County, people like teachers and school nurses were obliged to report serious physical abuse cases involving children under their responsibility.

Once the school nurse had found me crouched in a sort of cubbyhole off the main school corridor, weeping silently. She asked me if there was some problem at home and said if there was, I should tell them about it. They would help me. She brought me into her office and told me to take off my shirt, then asked where those welts on my back and shoulders came from. From a fight with a kid after school, I replied—probably not very convincingly, as part of me longed to share the whole story. Then I remembered how upset Mommy had been when I told her about the inquisitive nurse, and she warned that the welfare authorities might take us away from her, separate us, and put us in another home or even in an institution.

My most terrifying memories involve watching my father beat my mother. He would usually lose his temper at meals. There was a pervasive cloud of anxiety at the dinner table as we all wondered what triviality might set him off. One special trigger for his rage was any defiance of his edict that we eat sauerkraut at nearly every dinner. To this day I can't abide it, but somehow it became important to him that we choke down the stringy, bitter, and repulsive vegetable—and finish the last scrap of it. If not, we would be beaten. His weapon of choice was a belt because, he once said, he didn't want to hurt his hands. He used his fists only on our mother. I suppose that was his demented way of imagining himself to be a good parent.

From a modern perspective, it would be easy to criticize my mother for not having been more aggressive in reporting him for child abuse to the school or child welfare authorities. But she was in a nearly impossible position, with four children and, eventually, a pregnancy with twins, and she had no independent means of support. No money, no education, no job prospects, if she needed paid work. She was in a relationship that was toxic, but it was still a relationship, albeit often a violently abusive one. There were even moments of love and signs of a real closeness between my parents.

There were always so many children around, with my younger brothers and sisters. One had barely emerged from diapers before the next one appeared. My mother tried to escape once, by returning to her parents' home in Jenkintown, Pennsylvania, with all four of her kids (the last two, boy and girl twins, were born later). But as abusers often do, my father begged and threatened and promised and finally persuaded her to return to California, which naturally she did, and naturally she became pregnant again, this time with the twins.

I remember him beating her with his fists while she was heavily pregnant with them, perhaps a month before their birth. She eventually left for good not long after they were born, went to her parents' home, and declared that from now on, I, her son, would be the "man of the house."

My father never paid her a dime in child support. After she managed to get a quick divorce, unusual in those days but not unheard of, he disappeared. She had no money, no training for an actual job. She had a high school education, which is to say she could read and write just fine, but she lacked any marketable skills, like typing or shorthand. So she worked as a clerk in various businesses but hardly made enough money to support six growing children. Government welfare was not generous. In my memory, our welfare package, before food stamps came along a few years later, consisted of a weekly box containing a foot-long brick of Velveeta-like cheese known as "government cheese." Grilled cheese sandwiches became the staple of our diet. When we ran out of cheese, we switched to mayo on toast.

There was never enough food. My brothers and sisters and I made a pathetic game out of it. We would fight to be the first one to the table. And we would fight for the food, all in good spirits of course, but with an edge of desperation, since all these growing children were hungry. Always with a little guilt, the older kids pushed the littler ones away from the serving bowls. To this day, people comment on how fast I eat, whatever is on the table. We lived in a small rowhouse, with my mother's parents and her sister June. Poverty always made me angry, but it did not make us unhappy as a family. The big celebration in our house was what we dubbed Pollyanna Day, or my mother's birthday, on December 29. Since we never had enough money to get everyone Christmas presents, we all pulled names out of a hat on Thanksgiving Day to determine the person we would give a gift to on Pollyanna Day. To this day, the family gathers on that day—at this point with all the children and grandchildren and even great-grandchildren, along with partners, spouses, boyfriends, and girlfriends. Nearly a hundred people attend.

The house was small and packed. While Jenkintown was a prosperous place—a rich town about ten miles north of Philly, where stockbrokers and businessmen lived—we lived in the poor neighborhood, home to the gardeners and cooks and cleaning ladies who worked for the rich residents, and sometimes teachers and policemen, store clerks and tradesmen. My brothers and I slept in the attic, which was set up like a dorm with our four beds lined up, side by side. On the second floor, my mother had a bedroom, as did her sister, and my two sisters shared another room.

So, we settled in Jenkintown, went to the local public schools, and somehow muddled through. I always took my role as the man of the house seriously. We managed as a family. We always did. From age thirteen I often worked two jobs, as an usher in the local movie theater and as a dishwasher and busboy in a restaurant, contributing my earnings—and sometimes the proceeds of thefts, gambling, and burglaries—to my family. It was all easy to justify, given my consuming rage at the injustice of our poverty. Living in a town full of rich kids only accentuated those feelings.

Working as a caddy at the Foxcroft Country Club—where I carried patronizing members' bags and endured their abuse when, as often happened, they blamed the caddy for their flubbed shots—was like pouring gasoline on a fire.

"AFGHAN PEDOPHILES GET FREE PASS
FROM US MILITARY, REPORT SAYS"
New York Times
January 23, 2018

On 5,753 occasions from 2010 to 2016, the United States military asked to review Afghan military units to see if there were any instances of "gross human rights abuses." If there were, American law required military aid to be cut off to the offending unit.

Not once did that happen.

That was among the findings in an investigation into child sexual abuse by the Afghan security forces and the supposed indifference of the American military to the problem, according to a report released on Monday by the Special Inspector General for Afghan Reconstruction, known as SIGAR.

The report, commissioned under the Obama administration, was considered so explosive that it was originally marked "Secret/No Foreign," with the recommendation that it remain classified until June 9, 2042. The report was finished in June 2017, but it appears to have included data only through 2016, before the Trump administration took office.

The report released on Monday was heavily redacted, and at least in the public portions it did little to answer questions about how prevalent child sexual abuse was in the Afghan military and police, and how commonly the American military looked the other way at the widespread practice of *bacha bazi*, or "boy play," in which some Afghan commanders keep underage boys as sex slaves.

"Although DOD and State have taken steps to identify and investigate child sexual assault incidents, the full extent of these incidences may never be known," the report said.

CHAPTER 2

It Was Only in the Family

Surprisingly, I have happy memories of my father, even though the ones from my growing up, the ones I share with my siblings and close friends, and those I talked about with my mother until her death, are mostly violent and terrifying. I can vividly see that long-ago me—I tend to think of him as Little Rodney—and picture him approaching our father submissively, chin planted well down his chest, eyes on the floor like some cur kicked by his master his whole life. I see Little Rodney trembling night after night, steeling himself for the beltings he knew would be coming, not even daring to look up at his mother for fear his father would shift his rage toward her.

In retrospect, I realize that I have borne a heavy responsibility as the custodian of those memories because, in a sense, there were no other witnesses. My siblings were too young to remember the height of his abuse—though they too suffered from it.

It is hard dredging up memories of him not being a monster, being fatherly or caring, but, as I said, there are a few. Going to the beach, for instance, or taking the family camping. My father was an experienced woodsman, comfortable in the wilderness, with pitching tents and cooking over a fire he built. We sometimes borrowed an RV or a Winnebago for the weekend, and he took us up into the High Sierra (a four-to-six-hour drive from our home) and to the area around Big Bear Mountain, only a couple of hours away. On those trips, he would find a trout-fishing spot at just the place where the streams came cascading down; sometimes there were waterfalls feeding the pools, and he had an uncanny ability to find them. Huge trout swam in the eddies.

Some other weekends, we would all squeeze into the family car—no seat belts required in those days—and drive to the beach. What happy memories I do have appear in my consciousness like black-and-white images, snapshots from the time. As the highway to the seashore crested to the last rise before the final descent to sea level, we all had our heads out the windows like a bunch of dogs, alert to be the first to smell the salt air, our signal that we were close. Once in a while, my parents would host canasta nights with two or three friends. The couples would sit at a tablecloth-covered card table, with its matching set of folding metal chairs, and play this complex game. Someone looking in at the window would see a normal family, with a father who didn't hit with a belt because he wanted to spare his hands.

After all, he needed those hands in his job as a garage mechanic. I'm sure he wasn't the most technically sophisticated one in the shop, but rather the person who changed tires, pumped the gas, or did the menial chores. He was constantly losing his job, probably because he couldn't control his anger or, worse, was suspected of abusing a child nearby. After he was fired, he would return home in the middle of the night and tell us to pack our things because we were moving. There were four of us kids then, and we sat silently in the car, destined to start all over again somewhere down the road.

On my eighth or ninth birthday, I was sitting in our front yard when my father came home. I never knew how foul a mood he would be in, or what imagined transgression he would punish me for. This time was different. He came home with a present, a fancy chemistry set. I was stunned at the extravagance. You're a smart kid, he said, and you should learn all this stuff. Someday you could be a scientist yourself. I opened up the set, and it was as if I had entered a small laboratory or discovered a treasure chest. There were two doors and several shelves that contained canisters, test tubes, vials, little bottles or jars, some chemical compounds, and even a small rocket. A book of instructions explained how to make certain things happen, especially loud, messy, smelly things. (This set would never survive scrutiny by the Consumer Product Safety Commission today.)

I can't say that my father set me on a professional path with this gift—although I was first a biochemistry major when I went to college—but it was a rare moment of spontaneous generosity. And this might have set me up for my lifelong passion for science. Oddly, I never wanted to be a science reporter or writer, although I like to think that an appreciation for the scientific method greatly informed my work as a journalist. Start with a hypothesis, then test it against the facts until you come to some approximation, at least, of the truth, the always unknowable truth. For all his monstrous flaws, my father did instill in me some ambition. Just by saying to me, It's a chemistry set, go become a scientist, he made me think differently about my future, and about who I was and what I might be able to do one day.

He also enlisted me and other neighborhood kids in the Civil Air Patrol, a Cold War–era volunteer organization set up by the federal government to send people out to report on any aircraft they spotted at night. This was a time, the early to mid 1950s, when especially in coastal states, the prospect of attack by Russian long-range bombers seemed frighteningly real. Far enough from LA to see the Milky Way, we scanned the starry skies, holding up silhouettes of American and Soviet aircraft to compare them with what we saw traversing the night sky; I think we mostly spotted commercial airliners and private planes, which we duly reported to CAP. But it was a thrilling responsibility. The pleasure of that memory and my exciting first glimpses of the magisterial Milky Way on those nights is, however, spoiled by my adult realization that my father may well have been using CAP as a way of finding and grooming eight- or nine-year-old boys—my age at the time—for his sexual abuse.

That was the grim, pathological, criminal reality of the man. Plus, the nearly daily temper tantrums that so often ended with him pulling his belt off, in a quick, smooth movement that ended with a sharp crack as he lashed his children on the shoulders or back.

The first time my mother left him, she returned with us to her family's place in Jenkintown. Following the depressing though classic cycle of an abusive relationship, he begged her to return. He was going to change, he promised; he needed her and wanted to be with his family. I have a good idea what those conversations were like because my mother recounted them to me in riveting detail during our nocturnal chin-wags. Most of the neighbors had a good idea of what was said as well, since many were listening in on the party line that connected the adjoining three-story rowhouses on our street in that Philadelphia suburb where we spent the summer and then the winter of 1958 with my mother's parents and her sister June.

Suddenly, my grandfather Russell Myers was housing and supporting ten in a home that had never previously accommodated more than four. I was then probably in the fourth grade. I don't know if it was the pressure of all us children pining for the warmer climes of sunny Southern California or her parents' displeasure at a full house that made my mother return to our father. Maybe she still felt the love from her first encounter with him, handsome in a James Dean sort of way in his starched sailor's whites, straight off his US Navy warship in 1946. He swept her off her feet then, and so it happened again after she left. As with so many tormented wives and sadistic husbands, he was able to persuade her to leave Philadelphia and come back to California, to him. It took him a year, but she finally gave in.

Naturally, he got worse, and she entered a new phase of being an abused wife, the one in which she was inclined to forgive and excuse his violent behavior. Matters came to their final crisis between my parents during my mother's fifth pregnancy, two years after we returned to California. My father had insisted that she have her pregnancy looked after by a crackpot friend of his. Lacking health insurance, my father probably assumed that his price was right. Tellingly, he did not discover that my mother was carrying twins until the seventh month, when she was so heavily pregnant that it became obvious. My father's abuse escalated when he learned about the twins—as if he blamed her for two more mouths to feed. I remember watching as he beat her with his fists and then with a belt as well. After she had the babies, my youngest brother and sister, the beatings continued while my mother was doing her best to just take care of all six of us, often putting herself physically between him and us to thwart or moderate his attacks.

Finally, after one particularly vicious beating, my mother went to the police, looking for help; she took me along and I remember the encounter vividly. They told her there was nothing they could do about it, they couldn't possibly make a case against my father for striking her unless he had beaten her so badly that he broke a limb or caused some other obvious injury, or death. Put simply, in 1960 California it wasn't considered a crime to beat your wife. The desk sergeant snapped at her, "We're not marriage counselors here."

But just at this moment, luck turned in her favor. A really kind policeman took pity on my mother. He told her that he would go outside the law and arrest my father on suspicion of some crime (I could well imagine what that would be). Her parents wired her money to make the trip home again; we went to the Western Union office in LA and then to the Los Angeles station of the Southern Pacific Railroad, buying five couch seats (the twins were young enough to sit on laps, mine and my mother's). For her it must have been a logistical nightmare, taking six kids on a three-day train journey to Philadelphia. For us it was high adventure, the dawn of our freedom from domestic abuse and terror. We had to change trains in Chicago, and as I descended to the platform there, I accidentally dropped my little sister on her head. I've felt guilty about that my whole life; the blow to her head was bad enough that we all had to troop off to a local hospital, where she was examined and doctors declared she had a minor concussion but would be fine.

Our father was almost entirely out of our lives after that. Turns out he married again and had five more children. He was eventually accused of abusing them, both physically and sexually. Years later, I heard that he had been arrested, finally. I unearthed a clip from the *South Idaho Press*, from Burley, Idaho. On page seven of the edition of Tuesday, November 29, 1994, right below a story on the importance of residents appearing at public hearings on clean rivers and streams in Idaho, was a brief story with the headline "Accused Child Molestor's Bail Set at $500,000":

SANDPOINT (AP)—A Sandpoint man accused of kidnapping and molesting an 8-year-old boy is being held in jail on a $500,000 bond.

Bonner County Prosecutor Tevis Hull on Monday called Ronald Nordland, 66, a "predator" who constitutes a huge risk to the public. He said he would not seek the maximum penalty of death for first-degree kidnapping . . .

Nordland has a prior history of sex-related crimes, Hull said. He pleaded guilty in 1979 in Sandpoint to one count of lewd and lascivious behavior with a 12-year-old girl, Hull said.

A second identical charge was dropped in exchange for the guilty plea, according to court records.

Nordland was placed on five years' probation and spent 120 days in the sexual offender program in the Orofino prison. He later pleaded guilty to second-degree burglary and was placed on three years' probation, Hull said.

Nordland said he did not molest the boy, who was accompanying his 12-year-old brother delivering papers on Saturday. He denied he was a danger to the community because the prior incident occurred within his family.

Items described by the two boys were found in Nordland's vehicle, proving the kids are not making up a story, Hull said.

"(You) are looking at an individual who goes out in our community and destroys our youth," Hull said.

"He denied he was a danger to the community because the prior incident occurred within his family."

Like I said, I'm a ruthless reporter, even of myself. I now know quite a lot about that sordid case in Idaho and Ronald James Nordland's burgeoning career as a serial pedophile. I was already a seasoned reporter when that Sandpoint, Idaho, case first surfaced, and I talked to the cops out there at the time.

Ronald, as a three-time convicted sex offender under Idaho's strict three-strikes-and-you're-out law for sex offenders, was sentenced to life imprisonment, with no possibility of parole. Plus, one of his sex attacks involved the kidnapping of a child, a capital crime, punishable by death in Idaho as well as many other states. That he escaped.

My father wrote me a letter from behind bars, asking for legal help. He thought this aid should come from our mother, who had protected his children from him. Despite the fact that she was impoverished, due to his failure to make any child-support payments, he suggested she could find him a "Philadelphia lawyer" with the help of her "high class family." Almost in passing he mentioned a detail that he, ridiculously, considered exculpatory—this in his own hand, and signed and dated at the bottom: the boy's penis was in his mouth willingly. His defense was consensual sex with an eight-year-old. The letter bore the return address of his cell number, his prisoner number, and his prison address in Sandhurst, Idaho. It is my sole keepsake from him. I kept it to show to my brothers, should they ever doubt how evil was the father they had luckily mostly never known and whose abuse they probably could barely recall, since they were so young when it occurred.

That letter was a chilling keyhole view into the twisted psyche of a casually evil man. He died in prison, an end too good for him. But it saved me the trouble of hunting him down and killing him, which I once set out to do, in 1973. With my reporter's skills and experience, it was easy to find where he was living in Riverside, California, only a short distance from my early childhood home in Fontana. But after a long motorcycle trip across the country with my girlfriend, who was riding pillion and sensibly doing her best to dissuade me from my mad plan, I finally decided against carrying out patricide. As I later joked, it would have been a poor career move. The authorities got to him, and he was safely behind bars for good.

For a while, my siblings and I tried to keep this information from our mother's grandchildren. I now have more than twenty nieces and nephews—my kids' twenty-plus first cousins, whose ages bracket those of my children and who mostly lived in the same Philadelphia suburban area. They were all extremely savvy on social media. The effort to bury that sordid news was predictably unsuccessful, and once word got out, it traveled fast. When we learned that the vile newspaper item from 1994 had been unearthed, we knew that soon everyone would know of it, and many of us decided to tell our own immediate families before they heard about it from their cousins. That led to many hard and painful conversations with our children about the grandfather they thankfully had never met. As everyone knows, the spawn of abusers are themselves likely to become abusers. While that truism is supported by statistics, it is hardly any single victim's preordained fate. Because my mother escaped our father, and because she was such an extraordinary parent, we managed to avoid being too contaminated by his evil nature.

So, there you have it. I am the son of a convicted pedophile and kidnapper who died in an Idaho prison, sentenced to life as a repeat offender thrice convicted of child sexual abuse against boys and girls—a vile and abusive human being. I am also the son of a working-class single mother of extraordinary fortitude and devotion, who was determined to protect her children from him, which she did at brutal cost to herself.

"DESPITE EDUCATION ADVANCES, A
HOST OF AFGHAN SCHOOL WOES"
New York Times
July 20, 2013

SALANG, Afghanistan—There is not an ounce of fat on the wiry frame of Abdul Wahid, and no wonder.

After he finishes his morning work shift, he walks 10 miles down mountain trails in northern Afghanistan to the first road, where he catches a bus for the last couple of miles to the teacher training institute in Salang. He walks back up the mountain another 10 miles to get home, arriving well after dark, just in time to rest up for his day job.

In his determination to formally qualify as a teacher, Mr. Wahid exemplifies many of the gains for Afghan education in recent years. "It's worth it, because this is my future," he said.

CHAPTER 3

Making My Mother Cry

In my teenage years, I was constantly in and out of trouble: fighting, petty thefts. I was threatened with reform school if I kept it up, until one day I went too far and made my mother cry. And that turned me around. My siblings and I all addressed our mother as Mommy, even through adolescence in front of our peers and long into adulthood. Then, nineteen grandchildren later, her name morphed into MomMom for us all.

There is an old saying that a certain expertise in playing pool is a sign of a misspent youth. I was one of the tough kids in school—smart, defiant, clearly angry but determined to make the best of where we were. And good enough at pool that for a while I made money hustling rubes on the tables in a pool hall concealed behind a curtain (betting on pool was classed as illegal gambling) at the back of a barber's shop and several times larger than the shop itself. It was located on Jenkintown's aptly named Division Street, the town's one-block Black ghetto. My mother got a low-paid job at a local bank, processing checks. We cobbled together a life with her meager income, weekly deliveries of "government cheese," later supplemented by food stamps, and, as soon as I was able, my varied little jobs.

For some reason, the government cheese was delivered by the pastor of our local Lutheran church—we were considered Lutherans through my father's Nordic roots, and this pastor decided it was his role to save our souls. He would bring the cheese brick on Sunday mornings and then insist we go along with him to church services. The quid pro quo was infuriatingly obvious and tainted by the way that the pastor was also obviously sweet on my mother. All of this fed into my lifelong rejection of Christianity.

I began working, or so my Social Security records say, at age thirteen. My mother would never accept money directly from me— she valued my autonomy and liked the idea that my industriousness might serve to launch me from our circumstances. But I would buy food for the family, or pay some bills, or get my siblings clothes or school supplies or little presents. Maybe our junky old car needed to be repaired, and that was on me. Something always seemed to come up. My mother and I had an understanding that I was there to help financially. But she always made it clear she wanted much more for me.

I've always had a strong work ethic. I would get up at 4 a.m. to deliver newspapers with an old Jewish guy named Lewin. He had a corner on the newspaper delivery market in the area, with stacks of the *Philadelphia Inquirer*, the now-defunct *Herald Tribune*, and the *New York Times*. The pay was good for a kid and the work was pretty easy. We set out before dawn in his World War II vintage jeep; I sat in the back, folding the papers into easy-to-throw thirds and plastic-bagging them in bad weather—fourteen hundred papers every morning. Feeding the folded papers up to him as he sped along. Lewin had incredible throwing arms and would seamlessly launch the papers out the left and right car windows onto lawns and stoops on both sides of the road along the delivery route. That started me out reading newspapers—I especially loved the old *Herald Tribune*. Although I certainly had a sense of being part of this enormous machinery that gathered, produced, and distributed the news, I never thought I would be much more than a minimum-wage cog in the distribution machine.

I was too busy to give it much thought. By the time I was about thirteen, I was juggling four jobs: newspaper delivery boy, golf caddy, usher at the Hiway Theater in Jenkintown, and dishwasher at the International House of Pancakes. At the movie theater, I figured out how to get popcorn for free out of the coin-operated machine, and I would make little bags of popcorn to give away to my friends. I was sneaking many of them in through the back door for a quarter a head. We would sit behind the screen, which meant we watched a mirror image of the movie—not a problem. I also would caddy at the nearby Foxcroft Country Club, where wealthy WASPs and Jews would engage in a kind of parallel play—no mixed games for them. The other caddies and I would get tips and sometimes hack around on the golf course; we could play for free on Mondays, though frankly I despised the sport. Since we existed in a cash economy, the real attraction was the caddy shack, where it seemed an endless game of poker was played from the spring until the late fall, when they closed the course. I got proficient at the card table and in the end I caddied only to get access to the caddy shack. I had started realizing there were easy ways to make good money.

At the Division Street pool hall I flowered as a pool player. I could run twenty balls on a table easily from the break. Because I was young, people naturally underestimated me, and I would play with a friend and throw the game, impressing all the guys around me with my ineptitude. Someone invariably stepped up, eager to steal a dollar a ball, sometimes even more, from this kid who didn't seem to know what he was doing. And then I would run the table. Just lucky, the other guys would say, and try again. By that point it would become clear that I was running a hustle, and my marks grew angry. I loved the risk, the feeling of mastery, and the joy of taking the piss out of people who thought they could bully or rip off a kid. I suppose all these qualities are part of my character. They served me well over the years.

You can't live in that world without becoming physically tough as well, so I started boxing seriously. I would go to North Philly gyms with an older friend who became kind of a mentor and guide to the city's underworld, all the underground discos in the North Philly ghetto, after-hours jazz clubs, and the bustling boxing gyms. When I got older and stronger, I would work out there and sometimes get paid as a sparring partner for some of the professionals, ten dollars a round, pretty easy money for four minutes of work. Naturally, as an adolescent boy without a father figure, whose own father was not exactly the role model anyone would hope for, I made my own way, figuring things out as best as I could. And I became a seasoned fighter. In one memorable match at Jenkintown High School, where I made good grades until I didn't, I ended up boxing Mr. Popularity, the quarterback of the football team. I beat him easily since he didn't know anything about boxing. In that match I learned something important: the winner is not necessarily the tougher boxer or the better athlete, but the smarter one.

Then the football player's friend, who was a star on the school wrestling team, decided to settle the score and fight on his recently humiliated friend's behalf. So he attacked me, and I realized I stood little chance against someone twice my size. Even as he was trying to get me in wrestling holds, I coldly thought about my situation and decided what to do to end the fight quickly. So, I made a right jab to his Adam's apple; I put my whole shoulder, hips, trunk, and legs into it, as I had been taught. That did the trick.

The guy was in terrific agony. I understood it was a dirty punch—illegal in boxing, but it did have the effect of giving me status at school. Years later, I learned, to my horror, from a doctor friend that such a punch is potentially fatal—thank god it wasn't that time—one of many times in my life that I dodged a bullet. Soon everyone was afraid of Rod, and lots of guys wanted to show they weren't afraid of Rod, so I got into many fights. I legitimately developed a reputation for being a dirty fighter. Soon I was again among the outcasts. My grades tanked. I was one of those kids who had to reach the absolute bottom before he woke up.

Fifteen-year-old boys are not known for their restraint or good sense. I suppose the best way to channel their feral instincts is through sports or a vigilant parent or mentor. But my sports were boxing, playing pool, and a random game of golf before playing cards in the caddy shack, and my mother trusted me to a fault. I was headed toward self-destruction by the time I was fifteen. My best friend then, Bob, was the biggest guy in the school and also came from a troubled family. Kids on the edge flock together.

Our adolescent relationship was intoxicating—a combination of best friends and partners in crime. (Having been in many war zones, I've seen that same dynamic among adult men.) How any of us survive our adolescent selves is one of life's great mysteries. I suppose Bob and I confided in each other the ways kids do, but our favorite activities were skirting the local cops and committing petty, and sometimes not so petty, crimes. We would burglarize warehouses and specialized in stealing rolls of copper wire, which are easy to fence and very lucrative. And since we were so smart (naturally we *knew* we were smart) we were often suspected but never apprehended.

But the cops eventually got wise to us, certain that we were behind these burglaries, and they kept their individual and collective eyes on us. At a certain point in our life of petty crime, Bob and I got caught and were warned that if we screwed up again—"Your last chance, boys" kind of thing—we would be sent off to reform school.

Stupidly, despite the warning we weren't dissuaded from siphoning gas from a parked car when the tank of our old car ran out. We had used up our last chance. The cops caught us again. We were disinclined to surrender to the judge on our hearing date. We thought we knew where that would lead. We weren't in police custody at the time, and we figured our best option—here is that fifteen-year-old male brain at work—was to cut and run. Who cares if there were warrants out for our arrest? We climbed into my old '57 Chevy, which I had restored from a total insurance write-off while working in a body shop near my home. And we started driving the twelve hundred miles to Miami Beach, Florida.

Somehow, with what little money we had, Bob and I managed to rent a room for about twenty dollars a week for the two of us in the low-rent northern part of Miami. We were almost giddy with freedom in a place that was warm and exotic and beautiful. One time, I went into a sporting goods store and decided that, given all the water around us, I wanted a pair of flippers. I said to my friend, "I think I'm going to steal these things." Bob asked if they weren't a little too big to steal, and I assured him that they weren't. "Watch me," I said. "I'll do it." I put the flippers on and walked out of the store wearing them. I just kept on waddling away.

Eventually, we got arrested for shoplifting, this time in a supermarket, unaware of that fairly new invention, the CCTV monitor. The cops asked us for our IDs—which would have established that we were minors—but we insisted we didn't have any. We also refused to give our real names, addresses, or parents' contact details, though we did admit to our real ages. So, a detective was assigned to figure out who we were and what to do with us. All of this exemplifies the adage that sometimes you can be so smart, you're stupid. The detective, who seemed sincerely kind, warned us that based on our physical size, they'd have to put us in "county," by which he meant the Miami-Dade County Pre-Trial Detention Center, mostly a pretrial holding center for adults. The detective encouraged us to come clean so they could confirm we were juveniles, and then we could go into the much easier juvie system.

We refused, and off we went to the Miami-Dade County jail, where we could rot with all the other hardened criminals waiting to face their day in court. The two weeks I was there were a horrible experience. I was nearly raped in the shower, and despite my boxing skills I was no match for the other guys, who were professionals by comparison. I somehow managed to avoid being sexually assaulted, but Bob and I both got beaten up routinely and lived in fear.

We had been away for nearly two months, and during the two weeks we spent behind bars, I had plenty of time to think. I wondered how my mother and siblings were doing, what they might have heard about me, and how sick with worry they must have been. I resolved that if I ever managed to get out of this mess, I would turn my life around. (I cringe at the cliché—both the emotional one and the literary one—but there is no getting around it.) There was nothing I wouldn't do to get out of that place and make sure I never went back to one like it.

One day Bob saw that the nice detective we'd previously encountered was walking across the jail yard and shouted to him from the window: "Hey, we're ready to tell you the truth." I weighed in as well: "My name is Rodney Nordland," I yelled, "and I'm ready to give you all my information." We picked the right guy to confess to—he saved our lives. He took down our details and was able to find a warrant for our arrest from the Jenkintown police and the Montgomery County Courthouse in Pennsylvania. He told us that if that warrant concerned us, he could confirm with our fingerprints and Social Security numbers that we were juvenile offenders.

Much to our overwhelming relief, the detective got us out, and we were transferred into the custody of juvenile authorities. We told them everything; most important, probably, was where we were from. In the end the Miami-Dade County juvie authorities worked out a deal with their counterparts in Montgomery County, Pennsylvania, to sentence us to five years' probation for petty theft and malicious mischief, plus restitution for anything stolen, which our public defenders recommended that Bob and I agree to. After that played out, they put us on a plane home to face the charges there.

It was my first-ever plane trip.

Airports were different in those pre-terrorism days—more informal, easier to navigate. When the plane landed, my mother and my sister Cynthia (I had always been particularly close to Cindy) were waiting for me on the apron, at the foot of the plane's roll-up staircase, and they were both crying. I was moved that they were present and were so hurt by what I had done. I knew that I had to go straight. I got off the plane and we all embraced, all of us crying as they kept repeating that they had no idea where I was until the call from the police. I had deeply hurt the people I cared for most in the world. My mother had been through so much on our behalf. She had trusted me, and in return I caused her anguish.

That probation continued into my college years, which is one of the reasons I defied all the peer pressure to do drugs and never so much as smoked a joint—one of only a few people in college in 1969–73 who could say that. I lived in terror of going back to jail. It was a basic redemption story, built of the towering love I felt for my mother and my sympathy for and knowledge of the ordeal she had endured and survived for me and all my siblings. I was lost and now was found; I was the bad boy who became the straight-A student the year after flunking out of eleventh grade, which I had to repeat.

The Turkish novelist and journalist Ahmet Altan is serving a life sentence in prison in his home country, allowed to see his children only occasionally and his writing, in theory, limited to short notes to his family and lawyers. Earlier this month, however, Other Press published the English translation of his memoir, *I Will Never See the World Again*, which was written behind bars, defiantly, and smuggled out to that world he will never see. . . .

Here it must be said that the title of Mr. Altan's book is the statement of a brutal fact, rather than a cry of despair. There is not a smidgen of self-pity in the memoir's 212 pages. What emerges is this: You cannot jail my mind, and you cannot shut me up. "I have never woken up in prison, not once," he writes. "I am writing this in a prison cell and I am not in prison. I am a writer." . . .

On July 14, 2016, Mr. Altan and his brother Mehmet, a professor of economics and a political commentator, participated in a television program hosted by Nazli Ilicak, a prominent journalist. The next day, there was a violent aborted coup against the government of Recep Tayyip Erdogan, which included an attempted assassination, the bombing of Parliament, and nearly 300 deaths. The Altan brothers and Ms. Ilicak were accused of sending a "subliminal message" to start the coup.

Ahmet Altan and Ms. Ilicak were arrested and both condemned to life in prison. (Mehmet Altan was ordered acquitted by a higher court.) Ahmet Altan has exhausted every appeal to higher courts, and Erdogan is entrenched in power. . . .

A prisoner of conscience enjoys a certain prestige—including literary prestige—that a writer on the outside doesn't. I wanted to know how Mr. Altan felt about it. I asked: "Will life imprisonment ultimately have been worth it, since it enabled you to create this book?"

His reply was refreshingly frank: "Here is my honest answer: Yes, it is worth it. I need to tell you two things about myself: First, when I don't write, I'm nothing, I'm very ordinary; there's no difference between my presence and absence. I'm a restless person. Writing protects me from my nothingness and restlessness. I need to write in order to protect myself from myself."

CHAPTER 4

Channeling Rage

When I was a teenager, I had three ambitions—one might call them "career goals" today, but that phrase would have made me recoil, had someone used it in my presence. First, I wanted to become a novelist, one of those socially aware writers like Émile Zola or Charles Dickens. I read Dickens fanatically in high school, and I think that I sensed in him the kind of simmering rage at the violence and injustices of the world that I too experienced. He, however, created characters and scenes that opened people's eyes, maybe could even catalyze a change somewhere in society. I imagined being a kind of muckraking novelist, perhaps in the mold of Upton Sinclair or John Steinbeck—but never imagined journalism as a career.

My second ambition was to drive a race car. One of my part-time jobs was working in a garage with a bunch of guys.

Instead, I pursued a more affordable option, an overpowered Kawasaki motorcycle, which I took down south and entered in the racetrack circuit in North Carolina. But, as with boxing, when among professionals I quickly discovered that I was a relative amateur; I was way out of my league. In one race, I reasoned that if the Ducati in front of me could take the corners at seventy miles per hour, so could I; it was only a matter of getting up the nerve. So, on the seventeenth one-mile lap in the hundred-mile race, I resolved to stay on the

Ducati's rear wheel, come what may. Unfortunately for me, nerve was never something I lacked, but I overestimated my skill and went into an out-of-control spin that sent me skidding down the track hundreds of feet on my leathers—those quarter-inch-thick protective clothes, which were shredded to bits. My bike was totaled, but by some miracle I was not seriously injured. Gathering myself after my brush with death, I decided to give up racing entirely.

Finally, my third career goal was to discover the cure for cancer. In retrospect, this ambition has an unusual plangency, given my current situation, but as a high school student the situation was simple: the biology teacher had taken me under his wing, and I was fascinated by biochemistry. This was more than a decade after Walter Crick discovered the DNA molecule, but there was a lot of discussion about a biochemical breakthrough that would cure cancer. It's interesting to me now, since being a cancer patient has defined my recent life, that even though no one in my family had, up to that point, suffered from cancer (my mother's death from cervical cancer was decades in the future), I fixated on finding a cure for it. The reason might have been as straightforward as my combined curiosity, ambition, and finely tuned antennae, which were highly responsive to the zeitgeist. The government had embarked on its "war on cancer" in 1971, and research money was pouring into the field. Maybe my interest began long ago, with a thread of connection to my father: his weirdly unexpected gift of a chemistry kit, his offhand remark that I was a smart kid and maybe I'd become a scientist.

But the interest wasn't only sentimental or opportunistic on my part. I loved the order of biochemistry, the mysteries that resided not just in the chemical processes that made our balsa wood rockets fly, but those that made living organisms function—the brains, the digestive systems, the five mind-blowing senses. All of which, by the way, I appreciate now more than ever, given how my fragile but resilient brain has had to adjust to my current situation.

When I was a senior in high school, I wrote a paper and, encouraged by my wonderfully inspirational biology teacher, Ted Sherba, entered it in the national science fair, where it won an award. This later helped me secure academic scholarships. I speculated "On the Migration of Chromatid Filaments During Meiosis" (one of the processes of cell division that precede mitosis) as a subject worthy of further investigation because it might be instrumental in causing cancer. I was hardly the first person to take note of this curious process and its possible relation to uncontrolled cell division, but I was possibly one of the few high school students to do so. I became such a biology teacher's pet that—this is a little unbearable to write—when Mr. Sherba was out sick that year, I informally took over his class and taught it for him briefly.

But to be clear: as much as I may have changed my behavior and become the kind of overachiever parents dream of, I was still fueled by pure fury at injustice of every kind, at my father, at my mother's poverty and predicament, at snobs in school, at the anti-Semitism around me, and at the privileged golfers at the country club. I wonder sometimes how much effort it took, in those days, for me to contain all this anger and not let it explode, shocking its target with my disproportionate reaction to whatever offense was the ostensible trigger. We spend thousands on therapy in order to free ourselves from repression, denial, and withholding—but in my case all three, in various measures, were critical to my survival. And in many ways, my rage was a critical ingredient in my success—in school and subsequently as a journalist.

As a smart kid from a decidedly non-intellectual home, once I settled down and changed course, teachers who saw promise in this former degenerate stepped forward to mentor me. Another of them was my English teacher, Miss Jenkins. I think both she and my biology teacher were fond of me personally, and for me it was a treat to have highly educated adult role models. My mother was wonderful in many ways, but not in that one. Everyone, I've found, loves a redemption story.

Miss Jenkins was the first person to look at my writing and notice a certain talent. I've had great editors and learned from impressive professionals, but I will always credit Miss Jenkins with teaching me how to write. She pushed me to think about writing as a craft, with choices to be made and structure to consider. She offered what I lacked in life—a strong intellectual center of gravity. She provided the discipline and sense of clarity about how to approach my work, how to truly engage with the process of writing, and even (always a challenge) the importance of editing one's own work. I learned how to diagram sentences from her, something rarely taught nowadays, which I still think of as an influential skill.

Aside from these intellectual pursuits, and the true awakening of my intellect, the most valuable practical skill I emerged with from high school was my typing speed. Noticing the high percentage of attractive girls who took typing, and the fact that there weren't any guys in typing class (in those pre-computer days, typing was a profession reserved for girls), I signed up. No romance rewarded my decision, but by the time the semester ended I could type more than a hundred words a minute, a speed compatible with the way that I wrote. I thought fast and could write well, and with the grammar and syntax courtesy of Miss Jenkins—oh the sentences we diagrammed—I had assembled a tool kit that would serve me well over many years.

During my senior year, my brother Gary got into an argument in the street with a policeman, who then attacked him with a billy club. What the cop did was both excessive and unjust, and I wrote a letter to the editor of our local weekly newspaper in Jenkintown, the *Times Chronicle*. I described, at great length and with telling details, what had happened and criticized the police for their arrogance and aggressive, irresponsible actions. To my astonishment, given the conservative community the paper served, the *Chronicle* actually published this high school student's two-thousand-word screed. More surprising still was that the mayor of the borough launched an investigation, and the cop was ultimately punished with suspension. And my brother Gary received an apology.

Miss Jenkins saw the piece, and after telling me that it was too long—she was right, of course—she then said that I should see this as a kind of lesson. I should think of channeling my anger, as I did in the letter, into my writing, into journalism. She assured me that I wrote well, and she knew that I had a checkered past as a street fighter and runaway, that I had been in jail in Florida and was apparently trying to turn things around. I also imagine that she had had enough experience with adolescent boys to appreciate that things might easily fall apart for me if I didn't have some kind of goal. (She wasn't right about that, actually; I would never put my mother through more suffering, that much I knew.) But still, for me, this whole experience was a revelation, a kind of "Paul on the road to Damascus" moment that decisively shaped my life. I realized that she was right; there was a way to vent my anger at the world that was not sociopathic, but socially productive. I could write my rage. Not only that, but doing so could result in some kind of change for the better. I could find the people who were like me, cowering from my father as a kid, or like my brother, smacked around by an irresponsible cop, or like my mother, abused by a violent husband and tormented by aggressive bill collectors and bigoted neighbors. I could find those people and tell their stories, hold the bullies to account—but could I make a living at it?

Still, when I went to Penn State on full scholarship, I majored in biochemistry, and any kind of writing life wasn't on my radar. I also wasn't completely ready to commit to leaving my family. I spent the first couple of years at Penn State's little Ogontz branch campus in Abington, just a bus ride and a short walk from my house in

Jenkintown. After a few months, frustrated by the ordeal of studying organic chemistry and bored with school, I figured that I should get involved in the yearbook, something I had done in high school. I wandered around, asking where the yearbook office was, and accidentally entered the offices of the campus newspaper. "I want to volunteer," I said. "Sure" was the reply, and only after this exchange did I realize I was now part of the campus's little weekly newspaper.

By the time I moved to the main campus a year or two later, I realized that I was much more interested in reporting than in chemistry, and I switched my major to journalism. I spent much of my time writing for the huge main campus's student newspaper, the *Daily Collegian*, which was completely student run, on both the business and the editorial sides. It published about thirty-two pages six days a week, so it had a sizable staff. I never ascended in the hierarchy of the masthead: I was a reporter then and remained one for the next fifty years. I covered breaking news around campus, and those days, in the late 1960s and early 70s, campuses were busy places, with nearly daily demonstrations against the Vietnam War. Some of these protests were enormous, skirting the edge of violence. I joined a lot of them but then realized that when I covered them, I had to separate myself from the movement. This seems so obvious now, but as a kid reporter, the lessons just kept adding up. Working on that paper really made me a journalist because I wrote every day, which is the best thing you can possibly do if you want to be a writer. There were editors and student editors who took their job seriously, and faculty advisers from whom I learned a lot. But what I grasped more than anything was journalism's power.

Two of my stories managed to trigger some controversy. One, an opinion column, attacked the "Jesus freaks" on campus, who were aggressive in their proselytizing and attempts to convert students into born-again Christians. My girlfriend at the time was Jewish, and she was angry about them—especially one group that presented itself as "Jews for Jesus." I too found their aggression contemptible, and my own annoyance gained extra propulsion from how she took offense. So, I began to write a screed attacking them, not only for their intrusive and undesirable presence, but, in for a penny, outrageously attacking the whole concept of belief in the virgin birth, which I found preposterous. I argued that this was just a way of camouflaging the fact that Mary had been unfaithful to poor Joseph. The result was that outraged Jesus freaks set fire to piles of *Daily Collegian* newspapers around campus, something the Philadelphia newspapers covered gleefully.

This was a period, as I said, of campus demonstrations and militancy, much of it long overdue. I was assigned to cover a meeting of the Black Student Union. White students were banned from the meeting, so I ducked behind a curtain to listen in. That's how I learned the union had plans to set Old Main, the campus administration building, on fire to bring attention to the cause of Black students on campus. This struck me as extremely newsworthy, so of course I reported on it and, of course, that plan was nipped in the bud. First, the Black Student Union lashed out at me, accusing me of using illegal or unethical means to cover their meeting. They then banned me from covering future meetings and also took some newspapers and burned them, which is always a big mistake.

This time the story made not just the Philly papers but also the national press, and I found myself in the uncomfortable position of being lionized by Republicans and other right-wingers. And condemned by Black Power advocates and activists. I realized right away that conservatives were using me for their own purposes, and the reaction of the Black students gave them an excellent excuse to vent their racist rhetoric. This gave extra energy to what I had reported. Soon I was being interviewed by a few newspapers and got a job stringing for the *Philadelphia Evening Bulletin*. Plus, they offered me an internship in the summer. (My first three bylines were misspelled: one was Ronald Nordland, which infuriated me because it was my father's name, and the other two somehow overlooked the first *d* in my surname, so the byline was Rod Norland.)

Because I was the first of the Nordland kids to get a college degree, Mommy and my brothers and sisters were determined to go to my graduation ceremony and celebrate my accomplishment. The tears of sheer joy and pride that welled up in my mother's eyes were a welcome contrast to her tears of anguish and worry six years before. I was officially launched, graduating from college with a full-time job offer at a major metropolitan newspaper—the *Philadelphia Inquirer*, the *Bulletin*'s morning competitor.

The *Inquirer* hired me, which was a great thing, except for that snag of guilt from the knowledge that my success had been built, at least in part, on the story about the Black students' group. Of course, I had written hundreds of others, but that scoop put me on the map, got me an internship and subsequently my job. As good a story as it was, I still felt as if the positive personal consequences were in many ways due to the enthusiasm of a group of bigots I despised. On the other hand, I thought it propelled me toward a position in which I could help even the score in the great battle between Us and Them, whoever "they" are. I realized this would, one way or the other, be my life's work.

Finally, had I foreseen the article's reception, I would never have backed away from that story—or most other stories, if they were important to do. I am a ruthless reporter, which is a point of pride for me, not a source of discomfort—no matter how often the expression "ruthless reporter" is used to criticize or even undermine journalists.

"'NUKES' CAN TAKE THE HEAT"
Philadelphia Inquirer
April 1, 1979

MIDDLETOWN, Pa.—This town of 9,800 persons and many taverns is home to most of the workers at the Three Mile Island nuclear power plant, but by late last week it was almost a ghost town.

Almost, but not quite. While thousands fled, the "nukes," as nuclear workers often call themselves, stayed and willingly worked long hours at "TMI," as they call the Three Mile Island plant, and afterward spent long hours keeping at least the taverns here alive.

To all appearances, the nukes seem like any other blue-collar workers as they line up at the plant's observation center, waiting to be taken onto the island in pickup trucks. They favor blue jeans and plaid hunting shirts, metal lunch pails and hard hats with nicknames affixed in letters made of tape. . . .

In the midst of what industry and government officials say is the worst commercial-nuclear-plant accident in history, some of the men have sent families out of the area with the other refugees. But the vast majority have not taken even that cautious step.

From all accounts, they have all stayed on the job.

CHAPTER 5

Zig When They Zag

When I walked into the newsroom for my first day as a reporting intern at the *Evening Bulletin* in the summer of 1971, I was working on the desk, so the staff could supervise me closely. Then I started doing rewrite, which basically involved taking the reporting and rough copy submitted by a reporter, usually by phone, and turning it into a story. Turns out, I was pretty good at that, a skill that was helped by the speed of my typing. Soon the *Inquirer* hired me, and after I graduated from college in 1972, I started my new job as a staff reporter on a major metro daily.

I arrived during a period of remaking the paper into a force to be reckoned with, jettisoning some old hacks there, both reporters and editors, who had become complacent and stodgy. They scoffed at the idea of journalists with college degrees and refused to recognize the arrival of women in the newsroom. Like all new hires, the women started out as copy clerks, whose job was to race around the newsroom, ripping copy, often a page at a time, from typewriters and moving it to the right desks. The old guys would yell "Boy!" when they finished a page and insisted on doing the same to summon the copy girls as well. Finally, we younger newcomers hit on the sensible alternative of just yelling "Copy!"

The sale of the paper to the Knight Ridder chain began a period of remarkable transformation, truly the golden age of journalism, there and in many other newsrooms. About twenty young reporters were hired—many from journalism schools like Columbia—and we made up a cohort of young, independent-minded journalists who helped revolutionize the paper. None of this could have happened, however, without the extraordinary leadership of the great editor Gene Roberts, who took over the paper in late 1972.

I was hired just before Gene arrived, and because of my speed, I was assigned to night rewrite, which may have been essential to producing the paper but was basically a dead-end job profession- ally. I knew I had to do some time there, the newspaper equivalent of paying your dues or eating your spinach, but I was also eager to get out and start real reporting on a real beat. One night, I came into work feeling the pressure of a deadline, and there was an older guy sitting at my desk. "Could you get the fuck away from my desk, please," I said (sort of) politely. "I'm on deadline." The man looked up and apologized. "Of course," he said, as he got up and moved to another workstation. Immediately a couple of other guys at desks adjacent to mine got up and started asking me, "Do you know who that was?" It slowly dawned on me that he was someone import- ant, but other than that, I was clueless. This was Gene Roberts, our new editor in chief, they explained. I was so embarrassed, and impressed that he was gracious instead of asserting his authority and humiliating me. Later he told me that he appreciated that I was so businesslike, determined to get my story done.

Gene Roberts was just forty when he arrived at the *Inquirer* in 1972 and had already worked at the *New York Times* as the national editor. Before that he had advanced along the usual trajectory for those who rise high in the profession: moving from a smaller paper in his home state, North Carolina, to a larger paper in Norfolk, Virginia, to a larger paper in North Carolina's state capital, Raleigh; then to a really large urban paper, the *Detroit Free Press*, and then to the greatest newspaper in the country, the *New York Times*. He had covered the biggest stories of the decade for the *Times*, from the Kennedy assassination to the Vietnam War. As a Southerner he brought special sensitivity to his coverage of the civil rights movement and even wrote a book about it, *The Race Beat*. So when he arrived at the *Inquirer*, he was given free rein to make it a great national newspaper, and he adopted that attitude with his reporters. He let us loose on the world, encouraging us "to zig" when all the other journalists were "zagging."

I had been at the paper only for a few months when Gene arrived, but immediately, the staff felt the change in the atmosphere, a sense that we were working at the best possible place for journalists, with a visionary editor and a publisher committed to investing serious resources in the operation. President Richard Nixon's forced resignation following the Watergate scandal was still more than a year away, so we hadn't been infected with the "gotcha" frenzy in investigative reporting that developed after that. Nor the way that journalism became a prestige career for a bunch of Ivy Leaguers. All that would come to pass in only a few years. I was in the last group of reporters who started working without the ambition of bringing down a president and becoming a celebrity. For us it was all about the work, about getting great stories and being smart about the way we reported and wrote them.

Gene finally moved me from night rewrite to the police beat, always the first step for a young and hungry rookie. I had a desk in the police headquarters, one of those brutalist-style buildings in the confusing shape of a figure eight. The notorious Frank Rizzo had recently resigned as police commissioner to run for mayor. There are too many Rizzo stories to mention here, but one of my favorites was when he was called from a fancy dinner party to break up an antiwar demonstration, which he did while still wearing his tuxedo, a huge billy club sticking out of his cummerbund. The picture was published from coast to coast. There was no such thing as excessive force by the cops when Rizzo was in charge. He had little use for journalists on the police beat, especially someone like me, who at the time had such long hair that when I braided it in a ponytail, it extended way below my waist. Every time Mayor Frank Rizzo saw me, smarting as he was from the *Inquirer*'s coverage of police brutality, he made a snide remark about my apparently dubious gender. That made it an especially sweet moment when his commissioner had to give me the police department's good citizen award. This happened because I had been driving through Fairmount Park and saw a young thug kick the front wheel of a bicycle out from under an old man. I chased the culprit down with my company car, pinning him and the stolen bicycle against a wall and holding him there till police arrived. I later testified at the mugger's trial, where the judge gave him probation on the understanding that he would enlist in the marines.

I mixed up reporting on the cops with stories about municipal elections and unusually lucrative bingo games at the local firehouse. As I looked through some of my old clips, I came upon a story from November 1974 about the rape of a young servicewoman and the trial of her alleged assailants. Given my family history, I had a special sensitivity about vulnerable young women and the gratuitously violent men who cross their paths. I also hated bullies, and the defense attorney in this case seemed to relish making this woman cry.

In this story, an eighteen-year-old female army private hitched a ride with seven of her fellow service members. Later, she was found by the roadside after having been gang-raped by two marines and two soldiers. I covered their trial, which turned out, as these trials often do, with Miss H. being the one who was cross-examined and found guilty of, as the defense attorney told me, being "a slut." The defense focused entirely on her sex life up to the point of the attack, including how she may have engaged in oral sex with other men. The legal theory, if you can call it that, was known as the "prior chastity defense," which was, as I wrote, "a standard defense in rape cases." It forces "the victim to answer questions about her past sex life." In other words, the men were considered innocent because, experienced woman that she was, she was clearly "asking for it."

As I reread my story now, nearly fifty years later, I was impressed with how my twenty-five-year-old self channeled my rage at my father, at all men who brutalized women, into my work. "If she had been stabbed," I wrote, "could the defense have quizzed her about the wounds and bruises she had received in the past? If her home had been burglarized, would the defense have been permitted to humiliate her concerning her habit of leaving the doors and windows unlocked? Of course not. Just as surely the issue of her previous sex life is only of prurient interest in determining if a rape occurred. It is a defense rooted in an era when chastity was enforced by both law and public opinion. Today it is enforced actively by neither, yet the prior chastity defense lives on, feeding lasciviously on the dregs of Puritanism . . . Justice was served piping hot. But it still smelled bad."

Whether in Bosnia or Kabul, Cambodia or Nigeria, Philadelphia or Baghdad, I always seemed to gravitate toward stories about vulnerable people, especially women and children—since they will always be the most vulnerable in any society—being exploited or mistreated by powerful men or powerful social norms. I have taken it for granted, really, that these were the stories that needed to be covered, and I had a duty to do that. What was the point of being a journalist if you didn't make hidden injustices visible? What I understood only later was how what I had witnessed as a child had determined what I did later. That my father's treatment of all of us, especially Mommy, was hidden from public view, that he managed to continue his life of criminal abuse relatively unscathed, at least within our family, enraged me. Like countless abused families, we were invisible. To bear witness seemed to me to be my job description—whether I was reporting on young female soldiers brutalized on the witness stand or boys mistreated in a juvenile detention home (my first big investigative story, about the Camden County Youth Detention Center) or bystanders at a suicide bombing. This work was a useful way, as Miss Jenkins had observed, of channeling my rage.

Gene was a constant source of support and inspiration. He made me want to do my best work, and he watched our backs whenever management might have gotten annoyed about something. As a police reporter, I had a company car complete with a police scanner, so I could track what was happening and sometimes even beat the cops to the scene of a crime.

The car came in handy several years later when a nuclear reactor on Three Mile Island began to melt down on March 28, 1979. Of all the nuclear accidents in the United States, this one still stands out as the most dangerous, with radioactive gases and iodine released into the environment. Three Mile Island was on the Susquehanna River, about ten miles from Pennsylvania's capital, Harrisburg, and a hundred miles from Philadelphia, Baltimore, and Washington, DC. So, if a serious event happened there, it could affect significant population centers. The story has become a familiar one. Early Wednesday morning the meltdown began, a few hours after reactor operators had tried to repair a cooling system blockage. The next day a banner headline ran across our front page: "Power Plant Leaks Radiation; Mishap south of capital." I didn't write the story, but the lede summed up what had happened: "Radiation was released yesterday within a 36-mile radius at the Three Mile Island nuclear power plant southeast of Harrisburg, after a valve broke about 4 a.m. in the cooling systems of the reactor. The interior of the plant was evacuated."

We needed to own this story, which had taken place in our own backyard. Gene immediately deployed twenty-five reporters and divided us into two teams. One would be doing on-the-ground reporting at Three Mile Island and the communities nearby. Gene figured that a police reporter was the best person to take the lead because in a strange way, that whole area could be considered a kind of crime scene. So, he put me in charge of the on-the-ground team. The other team was in charge of the policy and science reporting—interviewing nuclear scientists and government officials.

Many reporters declined to go to Three Mile Island, for fear of exposure to radiation—especially younger people who had not yet started families. Our editors counseled each of us that no one would hold it *against us* if we decided not to go. Of course, the converse was also true: no one would hold it *for us* unless we did go. Looking back, I suppose I still had the illusion common among teenagers and young men: that they are immortal. If it weren't for that, how would you persuade anyone to jump out of airplanes or ski off cliffs or ride motorcycles at seventy miles per hour around corners? Or voluntarily go off to fight in a war? Or, for that matter, voluntarily go off to report on wars? No, back then, like so many of my peers, I just didn't believe I actually could die. The reality check would come later, somewhat spectacularly, but at the time it was an important lesson still waiting to be learned.

At Three Mile Island one of the first things I did was go to the reactor's parking lot and, with our team, take down all the license plate numbers on the cars parked there. I used my police contacts to (possibly illegally) obtain the home addresses associated with the license plates, and then my team and I used a criss-cross, or "reverse directory," to look up an address and from that locate the phone number and the name of the person associated with it. We divided up all the addresses and called every one of those people until we found some workers willing to talk. There will always be someone who wants the truth out. If you ask ten people or maybe twenty, you'll find at least one truth teller—and all you need is one. One will always know others, or lead you to them.

The ones we found told us that despite the utility company's assurances that things were under control, the situation was in fact much worse than anyone outside the plant knew. My police scanner, which is a radio, made it possible for me to scan all the frequencies of the walkie-talkies inside the plant. I listened to people saying, "Oh my god, this is out of control. What are we gonna do? We're gonna have a meltdown."

This was what I was born to do: get fully immersed in a gigantically important story, work with and direct a team, dive into my own reporting, and find my own stories. I don't remember bothering to sleep much, except possibly in the car; the adrenaline and the sense of purpose made sleeping feel like a waste of time. And for once, I wasn't preoccupied 24/7 with my latest love interest. By the following Monday our team had produced a huge report about the incident, delving into the inner workings of the reactor, the community surrounding it, the residents who had to decide whether to remain in the area or leave. A few days later I broke a story revealing that the Nuclear Regulatory Commission had misled the public when it said that no leak had occurred. I don't know how many stories we finally published. But no one reported this national news event better than the *Inquirer* under Gene Roberts. Our Three Mile Island coverage won the Pulitzer Prize in Local General or Spot News Reporting.

Gene was impressed with my work on Three Mile Island, but even so I was unhappy at the time. Many months before that story broke, Gene had brought me into his office, and the meeting was not what I had expected. He said he wanted to move me to cover suburban Philadelphia, specifically the Main Line suburbs in Delaware County. Here I was, this hotshot police reporter, assigned to covering school board meetings on the Main Line. I sat in his office, incredulous and upset. How could there be anything out there worth covering, compared to Frank Rizzo's brutal cops? But Gene was always playing chess while the rest of us were playing checkers—thinking many moves ahead.

He explained that the battle for newspapers then was in the suburbs. The paper had to win there to survive. Big metro newspapers were getting their asses kicked by small suburban newspapers; white flight was destroying cities and eroding our subscriber base because people wanted to read about school board meetings and other local happenings we didn't cover. "I want you to go out there and cover school boards like a real journalist," he told me. "And a real journalist will find a story anywhere, and you can do that." He felt that I could generate stories that would bring in suburban readers, who would be the paper's future; advertisers would happily follow. He acknowledged that this assignment would not provide the kind of fun that I had been having, but he promised me this: "One day, I will reward you for this. And I always keep my promises."

I understood his logic and said that of course I would do what he asked. But for the first time in my life, I drafted my résumé. The battle for the suburbs was ultimately one the big city papers, even one as good as the *Inky*, would lose. We all knew that, probably even Gene did—but he also had other moves in mind.

One of those moves started to play out seven months before Three Mile Island, when the pope, Paul VI, died on August 6, 1978. No one could have known it then, obviously, but it was the beginning of an extraordinary period. There would be three popes in as many months.

Gene called me. "Do you have a passport?" he asked.

Of course I didn't have a passport. Why would I have a passport? A suburban Philly ex-hoodlum who had never been on an international flight, or to any other country except Canada, which I went to by car.

He told me to get one as quickly as I could because he wanted me to cover the death of the pope and the naming of the next one like no one had ever covered the Vatican. Find some great stories, he told me. Zag when all the hacks zig.

Within days, I went from covering school boards on the Main Line—and yes, I had already broken a great story involving the Warlocks motorcycle gang and a school board president, but that's for another time—to being a foreign correspondent.

"IN BAGHDAD, WHERE 'HELLO' MEANS GOODBYE, HELLOS ABOUND AT TRAVEL AGENCIES"
New York Times
June 13, 2014

BAGHDAD—Iraqis say "hello" when they mean goodbye. This can get a little confusing to visitors who do not speak the local dialect of Arabic and think they are hearing English, instead of a borrowed word that has been inverted in meaning.

There were a lot of hellos on Friday at the travel agencies lining Sadoun Street here. Normally, they would be closed on a Friday . . . Even the celebrated Icepack, an ice-cream parlor that is normally mobbed on June weekends, when temperatures already reach well into the 100s, was closed.

The travel agents, though, were open, and busy. "It's a rush, really a rush," said Haider al-Rubaie, the manager of an Iraqi Airways travel agency, as he juggled telephones, customers, and carbons of actual air tickets, which are still common here. "Some days they're adding eight flights, when the usual is one or two."

Asked where the passengers are heading, Mr. Rubaie shouted, "Anywhere!"

"Any country that doesn't need a visa, they don't care where they go, just so they can leave," he said.

CHAPTER 6

Dividing the World

I'd never before been to a foreign country. But for me, arriving with
a job to do instead of as a tourist made everything easier. It turned
out that the skills and instincts I had developed as a metro reporter
in Philly could easily be redeployed as a foreign correspondent: getting the lay of the land, befriending people on the inside who knew
what was going on, keeping my eyes open for things that struck me
as strange, or wrong, or just interesting. And for the next fifty years,
in war zones and in jungles, in sophisticated urban neighborhoods
and in godforsaken communities, in areas under active bombardment and those that were counting and stacking their dead, these
approaches worked.

Shortly after I arrived in Rome, I met two reporters from the
Catholic News Service who covered Rome and the Vatican and knew
the scene intimately. I met them in the Foreign Press Club of Italy,
where we reporters transmitted our stories from the telex machines.
Because I was a good typist, I was tapped to punch telex tape for
nearly everybody there. I quickly filed a few Catholic News Service
stories for its reporters, and a friendship developed. The first night
we were supposed to meet for dinner, they suggested that I meet
them at some trattoria—which I had assumed was the restaurant
name, instead of the Italian word for "restaurant." That evening,

I went to the Via del Tritone, one of the main drags in the center of Rome, looking for a restaurant called the Trattoria. I asked some people for directions, and finally they just started laughing, much to my embarrassment, as they explained to me the reason for my confusion.

As everyone was preoccupied by the funeral preparations, then the burial, and finally, the papal conclave where the cardinals were tasked with selecting the next pontiff, it became clear to me how many news stories weren't getting covered. I was fascinated by the debate about abortion, for instance. This devoutly Catholic country was on the verge of legalizing it and making family planning broadly accessible. These kinds of stories would resonate with readers back home because the abortion debate was front and center in America, and Philly was a heavily Catholic city.

Once the conclave was over, a new pope, John Paul I, was chosen on August 26, and a few days later I returned stateside. Back to the school board beat on the Main Line. But no sooner had school started than John Paul I had a heart attack and died, so the paper sent me right back. I ended up spending several months in Italy, covering the popes and other stories. And by that point, I had gained a taste for being a foreign reporter, working in a language I didn't speak and seeing stories everywhere. I loved the work and wanted to keep doing it.

When I returned home, I reached out to Gene Roberts. He was famous for his unusual interviewing approach, which he also used in meetings with staff. Apparently he developed this when he covered the South during the civil rights era for the *New York Times*. He would approach sheriffs when they were banning marches and brutalizing protesters or call them up, introduce himself, and just wait, without saying a further word or, at most, asking a simple question. After hearing the answer, he wouldn't say anything, so inevitably the person he called or met with got unnerved and started talking and talking and talking some more. They would take the lead and steer the conversation into rich and unexplored areas, providing insights and quotes that would never have surfaced during a conventional interview. (Gene attempted to use this technique with one reporter who was determined not to submit, and they sat in silence on the telephone for half an hour. Gene spoke first and said, in his lazy Carolina drawl, "Well, Jim, it was sure nice talking with you." And then he hung up.)

So when I called him and said, "Look, I want to keep doing this kind of work," Gene said nothing. Naturally, I started babbling away, saying, "Gene, I really want to be a foreign correspondent. I really love this work. I know I don't have language skills, but you know, I can gain them and I think I'll be good at it and I promise to zig when everybody else zags just as you always ask." And even though I left him little room to interrupt, I knew that he never would, that he would keep letting me twist in his silence. I figured I may as well fill it up and make my case. Finally I finished, and after a long pause he said, "Well, stay tuned to this channel. Something may happen. Just keep doing what you're doing. We'll find something for you."

It wasn't long before Gene asked me to visit him at his home, a lovely townhouse in the Old City of Philadelphia. It was entirely decorated with Asian art. Gene himself had been a foreign correspondent, in Saigon for the *Times*, and he had become a serious collector, especially of art depicting early encounters between East and West. He started telling stories about his career as we sipped some cocktails, and finally, he got around to the point.

He told me he wanted to build a foreign staff. He had already sent out another young reporter, the brilliant writer Richard Ben Cramer, and assigned him to a base in Rome. From there Richard would cover the world east to Afghanistan. Then Gene told me that he wanted me to do the same kind of reporting I had done in Rome, but based in Bangkok, Thailand, and from there, I would cover everything east of Afghanistan.

"So, when you get there," he said, "you really got to kick ass. You know, I have confidence in you. And I think you will."

And I then said what I knew he was about to say: "Yeah, I get it," I said, my excitement mounting. "I should just zig when everyone else is zagging."

He deployed me to a region that he knew well. Eleven years before I went to Thailand, Gene spent a year covering the Vietnam War for the *New York Times*. He understood how the effects of the war lingered and had spilled out all over the region, but while he was a brilliant reporter and editor, he didn't take to being a foreign correspondent. He served his time, checked that box, and returned home to move into important leadership positions in newsrooms like those of the *New York Times* and the *Inquirer*. He must have seen something in me that made him realize I was different. That this life of wandering around different foreign countries, where I didn't speak the language or know the culture but managed to find stories, was the work I was meant for. The only evidence he had that suggested I might succeed was my performance during the short parade of dead popes in Italy. But, as it turned out, this was enough.

That's when my work life really began. On October 30, 1979, an article I wrote from New Delhi on the Hindu new year had an italicized note at the top: "Inquirer *reporter Rod Nordland wrote this article in India last week before flying to South Korea to cover the assassination of President Park Chung Hee.*"

Yes. I knew I would never do anything else. Who would want to?

"WHERE FEMALE ELEPHANTS WITHOUT TUSKS ROAM—AND POACHERS STAY AWAY"
New York Times
June 16, 2018

ADDO, South Africa . . .

Addo's rangers tend to get emotional about their elephants. Michael Paxton, the ranger, took visitors to the final resting place of a big tuskless cow who was accidentally injured in March trying to force her 12-year-old son out of the herd, a normal social behavior.

The young bull resisted forcefully, breaking his mother's leg so badly a bone protruded and rangers had to put her down. As soon as that happened, elephants that were scattered around the park—every one of them probably a relative of some degree—started coming to the body.

Some came from as far as 20 miles away until scores were standing nearby, their heads hanging, either quietly or making a low rumbling noise, in what some zoologists have interpreted as a display of mourning.

Mr. Paxton pointed to the elephant's bleached skeleton, picked clean by scavengers.

"They still come to visit here," he said.

"They're so incredibly intelligent," John Adendorff, the park's conservation manager, said. "They cuddle their young and spank them when they misbehave. But I hate to say that they're close to humans, because we're the scourge of this planet. They're not."

CHAPTER 7

Only in Africa

Some of the most fun I've had as a journalist has happened during trips to Africa. Something about the place just brings out the juvenile delinquent in me—in a good way. It's always a challenge working in Africa. And almost always, the first challenge is just getting in (which, aside from a few tourist-friendly countries like Kenya and Botswana, can be daunting). For instance, Sudan and Darfur Province don't make it easy. The photographer Gary Knight and I spent pretty much a year lobbying Sudanese officials for a visa just to get into Sudan, let alone into the troubled Darfur region. And that region later would be the scene of a genocide committed by the Janjaweed militia, which worked at the behest of the Sudanese government to carry out mass rape, murder, pillage, and other crimes that later would be classified and prosecuted as war crimes (genocide and crimes against humanity) by the International Criminal Court in The Hague. Charges like that were eventually brought against President Omar al-Bashir of Sudan, who for many years was unable to travel to certain countries in the West for fear of being arrested and taken to The Hague to face those charges. So just getting a visa for a journalist to enter Sudan had not been possible for years. The authorities there were especially sensitive to issues related to Darfur. I remained determined to get in, flying to Paris when I heard the Sudanese foreign minister was there, so I could try to get a meeting with him, or ambushing him during a UN General Assembly speech in New York. At the time I worked for *Newsweek*, with an unlimited travel budget (business class for flights over two hours, first class for those over six) and a great, tactically useful feature called the back page, to use as a bargaining chip. The last page of the magazine's international edition was reserved for a Q&A with some prominent official, which was published verbatim. Officials loved it because they knew that it would not be edited, that it would be exactly their words, as they spoke them, lies and all, whatever. It helped in gaining access to officials. So, I basically arranged a barter: to get visas for Gary and me, I traded the back page of *Newsweek* through the offices of Sudan's foreign minister. It was a fair deal. He got his opportunity to spew his views, unedited, and Gary and I headed for Sudan.

Then we faced the problem of getting into the Darfur region. We did somehow manage to do that, after lots of meetings with junior officials in Khartoum, the capital of Sudan. And with the help of fixers, of course. After several days of trying, Gary and I secured the permit allowing us into Darfur Province, which is the size of France (Sudan is one of the biggest countries in Africa). When we drove up to the internal border, the officials at the checkpoint took a look at the piece of paper granting us permission to enter. They threw the paper in the dirt, saying, "This is no good here. Journalists are banned from Darfur." Then the officials turned us back. So I picked up the paper, then a bit worse for wear, and kept it. We managed to find the unit of the African Union peacekeeping force (African Union Mission in Sudan, or AUMIS) that had been sent to Darfur to try to keep the peace and restrain the excesses of the militias, especially the Janjaweed group. So, Gary and I talked to members of this unit and persuaded them to take us along on board the ground vehicles and planes that accompanied their troops; they accepted our paper as valid and either did not know or chose not to know that journalists were banned. We got into Darfur that way and managed to get away with remaining there for a good week or more. I knew, of course, that our stay would last only until my first dispatch datelined "Darfur, Sudan" was published, so I had to make it a good one. I wrote about the wave of horrific assaults on international aid workers in the Darfur region.

That dispatch was transmitted from Darfur and, as we later learned, intercepted immediately by the authorities. But the piece was published only in part in *Newsweek,* with the sexual assault material left out due to editors' concerns about anonymous sourcing and the worry that there was enough detail in the story to possibly indirectly identify victims. But the authorities saw the original. Soon government radio was broadcasting Gary's name and mine, announcing that two American journalists had illegally entered the region. Not for the only time, I was effectively a fugitive from injustice. Our African Union peacekeepers expressed regret but said they could no longer host us, and we had to leave, finding our own way out to the Sudanese capital, Khartoum. We no longer worked outside in plain view but stayed behind closed doors as we made our way to the capital and its international airport.

After getting into Darfur when no one else could, I got an email from a colleague with the *New York Times*: "Rod, how'd you do it? How'd you get into Darfur? Can you tell me what I need to do?" We journalists who cover wars and other conflicts make up a fairly small community. We all know one another; we meet in one war or other crisis after another. We're very competitive, but not when it comes to sharing information about how to get into and move around in certain places because that's how we figure out how to stay safe. And we're always willing to help one another in most cases. A big exception at that time was the *New York Times* journalists. As was often said, they always take but they never give. They were notorious for being that way, but that has changed a lot in recent years. And I'm glad to be part of that change. And there are a lot of *New York Times* colleagues who are great about sharing.

Anyway, in this instance, the *New York Times* journalist emailed me and asked me to share my contacts and tell him what you had to do, once inside the country, to get a permit to enter the Darfur region. And so I shared all that with him.

And then, a few years later, Darfur was back in the news when President al-Bashir of Sudan was charged with war crimes by the International Criminal Court at The Hague. And so journalists were trying to get back in, and it was completely impossible. Gary and I were by then marked men, and there was no way we could return. But one of our colleagues did—the one I had helped before, so I emailed him and asked him how he did it.

I had no answer from him. Then, a year later, I got into Somalia, when that had become very difficult to do. The country was then being run by what were called the Islamic Courts. These Islamist militias brought order to a very chaotic, lawless place and imposed some sort of peace. And that created a moment when it was actually possible to get into Somalia safely by enlisting the protection of the Islamic Courts; at many other points in recent history, such a thing was not possible. This was when I heard from that colleague again, the one whom I had asked to return my favor. He had never answered my email asking how to get into Somalia and Darfur. By now I'd figured out how to make contact with the Islamic Courts there and managed to get in. Actually, I flew in on a plane with the World Food Program, which was pretty friendly to journalists; the organization wanted people to know how dire the famine in Somalia was at that time. So I found my way in at a time when, for a while, no other journalists did. And this same journalist colleague wrote and said, "Rod I'm sorry, I just now saw your email. I missed it when you sent it to me [a year earlier]. And oh, by the way, how did you manage to get into Somalia last month, could you tell me what I need to do?"

I was tempted not to tell him, but I have always believed that I should do everything I can to help my colleagues stay safe. And most of them do that for me too, with the exception of that *New York Times* colleague.

On another trip into Somalia in 2008, I had a wonderful only-in-Africa moment. On one occasion, I went deep into the west of the country, where a provisional government had set up its headquarters in a town called Baidoa, kind of the epicenter of the famine and close to the border with Ethiopia. A group of foreign journalists, including me, were staying in the house of an Irish refugee aid group, who were kind enough to give me shelter. The area was overrun by warlord groups, who were less organized than the Islamic Courts and unfortunately were pretty much all stoned on khat, a narcotic plant consumed by chewing. Many of them kept a cud the size of a medium apple in their cheek. Now these stoned militiamen had surrounded our compound and were firing into its mud walls.

Half a dozen journalists were in the compound, and one of the Somali Islamic Court militias was there, guarding it. And they got up onto the walls and started firing over the warlords with their AK-47s. Then they began passing out AKs to journalists, asking us to help them lay down more covering fire to protect the compound walls, making it less likely that we would be overrun. I thought briefly about doing this, but I've always abhorred the use of firearms and I believe the Geneva Conventions actually dictate that journalists cannot serve as combatants. And as soon as you pick up a weapon, you're a real combatant, never mind the circumstances. So I passed, but some of my friends didn't. And in the end, the problem went away. I guess the warlords had other people to terrorize or other responsibilities that day.

Getting into Somalia meant hiring what they call a technical—a pickup truck with a machine gun mounted on top of the cab, or sometimes on the bed of the truck. Half a dozen armed men on board serve as your bodyguards and take you to appointments and so on. The men on the technical were frankly terrifying. They were routinely stoned on khat, and as is the case when people abuse drugs or alcohol, adding guns to the mix can be toxic. Our technical would meet us journalists at the Mogadishu airport—no terminal to pass through or formalities to exchange. They just drove right out onto the runway tarmac and pulled up to the stairs by the plane. The first stop would be the Hotel Shambo in downtown Mogadishu, a building that had been shot up and shelled so much, rubble from smashed concrete was everywhere, and the hallways and rooms had a coating of dust and dirt an inch deep. It was amazing that the building, or rather three or four floors of it, was still standing. The Shambo did have one virtue: an accessible flat roof. Though it was deep in dirt, the roof was perfect for setting up satellite transmitters, which connected journalists to the internet. If you had a room on an upper floor, you could snake a long cable from the BGAN satellite transmitter down through the window of your room and connect your computer—the Shambo had no air conditioning, so keeping the window open was not a problem. (I'm not sure the place even had hot water.) On really hot nights we'd spread a ground cloth on the roof and sleep in the relative coolness up there, on a mattress of fine dust. On that trip, I had heard that refugees had taken to renting trees from farmers as shelter from the fierce sun.

There is a good general principle for reporters trying to get a leg up on an important story: *Cherchez le misérable.* In 2008 Zimbabwe was facing a historic election. For the first time there was a serious opposition challenge to the then fifty-year rule of Zimbabwe's autocratic president, Robert Mugabe.

His popular challenger, Morgan Tsvangirai, was clearly poised to give him a good run in the upcoming elections. That would possibly mean toppling the last of the African Big Men, those dictators who emerged from the continent's decolonization: Idi Amin, president and cannibal-in-chief of Uganda, and the CIA stooge Joseph Mobutu in the Congo, whose epic corruption made him one of the world's wealthiest men, ruling one of the world's poorest and saddest nations.

So Zimbabwe's 2008 election was bound to be big news.

The Zimbabwe government responded by clamping its borders closed to foreign journalists, denying them visas, and publicly announcing that no foreign journalists would be allowed to visit the country during the election period. But because the economy depended on tourists, they couldn't really prohibit all visitors. Tourists, however, needed visas, and Zimbabwe's embassies routinely demanded to know each visitor's profession. *Newsweek*, like many news organizations then, had a policy requiring that its correspondents not falsely represent themselves, claiming to be something they were not. My personal work-around: I put down my profession as "media worker" or some other vague euphemistic term.

There would still be the problem of moving into and around Zimbabwe undetected.

Unfortunately, I happen to look like a journalist, and pretending to be a tourist never works for me. So I reached out to an opposition politician, one of the country's persecuted white farmers and a representative of that community. Their lands were being confiscated, then given in small holdings to poor Blacks, especially ones who were members of Mugabe's ruling party, the Zanu PF. That pretty much resulted in the destruction of Zimbabwe's once prosperous agricultural sector. Small holdings are just not capable of large-scale production. They were better adapted to subsistence farming, so *le misérable* in this case was the white farmer. I won't name the one I reached out to, as Mugabe's party is still effectively in power even if he's not.

This man introduced me to something called Hushmail and then insisted we exclusively use that early platform of heavily encrypted email.

We communicated that way, and he gave me instructions on how to enter the country safely: through the southern province of Bulawayo, bordering Botswana and South Africa. Bulawayo was a stronghold of white farmers, and from there they put me on a sort of underground railway, from one white farmer to another, until I reached the capital, Harare. When I settled into the Meikles Hotel, the staff immediately figured out that I was a journalist, of course, especially when I asked for a southern-facing window. This was so I could deploy my BGAN satellite internet transmitter, which needed to reach the satellites generally in the Southern Hemisphere, well south of Zimbabwe.

The BGAN transmitters can reach satellites and connect to the internet from pretty much any place on earth. You just need a good line of sight from your window or roof to the satellite's position in the south, which you can detect with a feature on the BGAN. Beeping grows stronger and faster as your aim at the satellite improves. Once the beeping becomes practically a continuous whine, you know you're logged on to the satellite.

The hotel staff were aware that I was doing this. They spoke in conspiratorial tones when giving me advice on how to move from the hotel without encountering the authorities.

And that approach worked for a while, until I rented a car to cruise around the city and came across an election rally downtown. A crowd of activists had noisily gathered around a police pickup truck. Officers were putting selected demonstrators and members of the crowd into the back of that truck.

When I stopped to talk to people in the crowd, they immediately took notice and accused me, correctly, of being a journalist. They tried to put me in the pickup. Some of those already held inside said, "Look, you should just jump out of here and run for it; you're a foreigner so they won't dare hurt you."

My car was not that far away. And to help me, the fast-growing crowd put themselves between the police and my car, and then between the police and me, as I ran to the car. And then between the police and my car as I jumped in and drove away—I told my Zimbabwean fixer to melt into the crowd and lose me; I didn't need a translator, as English was spoken pretty universally, and he would have been far more vulnerable to official reprisals than I was.

In my rearview mirror, I saw that the police had taken off in immediate pursuit, heading toward me in their truck.

That was the first time, and probably the last, that I actually was involved in a police chase—another of those only-in-Africa moments. Somehow that mysterious African jungle telegraph was working impressively well in Harare that day.

News of my police chase spread among groups of people along my path. As I drove, crowds got in the way of the police to slow them down. Others directed me into a side street or an alleyway and then filled the street behind me.

This went on for something like half an hour. If only I had had a dashcam or an iPhone back in those days—the flow of the route and the people was incredibly cinematic. At one corner the bystanders signaled me to turn onto a side street—but it dead-ended in a park on the corner, so the only way to get to it was to plow through the bush and turf of the park and bounce over a couple of curbs. I was immediately reminded of that old joke:

Q: What's the best all-terrain vehicle?

A: A rental car.

I was in the midst of a huge, good-natured conspiracy of regime haters, who laughed uproariously at my vehicular antics and at the police's pathetic attempt to catch me.

The officers did not try to shoot me. Fortunately, they never opened fire on my car or even threatened to do so. I'm sure I would have stopped in that case, the risk-versus-reward calculation tipping the scale toward giving myself up.

Luckily, as often happens for journalists, the authorities are aware that shooting one of us would be really bad PR, so they restrain their violent instincts.

So I felt reasonably safe in that car chase. Soon my vehicle was alone in the streets, and I managed to get back to my hotel. Then I went on foot to find a place to file, which happened to be an internet café in a shopping center.

The whole thing was, frankly, great fun. And also a convincing demonstration of the collapse of Mugabe's popular support.

I was kind of thrilled by it, to be honest.

The rest of my time covering that election was similarly cloak-and-dagger, and everywhere I felt protected by the seemingly widespread support of the populace. I often noticed Mugabe's Men in Black—intelligence agents from his Central Intelligence Organization who were following me, eavesdropping on me at the internet café or when I tried to do voxpop (man in the street) interviews. They were easy to spot, quite comically dressed in worse-for-the-wear black suits, threadbare in places, ill-fitting but freshly pressed. These agents were also sporting a yellow tie or a yellow carnation in their boutonniere. If that wasn't enough to make them obvious, other Zimbabweans were constantly pointing them out to me.

I filed the resulting *Newsweek* story from the internet café instead of the hotel roof, which unfortunately wasn't flat, and trees blocked the south-facing windows of the room. I left out the car chase, worried that the rental car company would pursue me for damage to their vehicle.

In those days, *Newsweek* kept a fully equipped Land Rover in Nairobi, and I was able on several occasions to use that and set up my

own safaris, hiring an Indian gentleman named Ahmed who was experienced at that sort of thing. He would pitch camps for our staff,
arrange cooks and trackers, and guide us along the way. My friend
Matthew Naythons and I camped with Ahmed and his crew in the
savanna of western Tanzania. And one afternoon we were surrounded
by a troop of baboons. Quite a large troop. Baboons are scary animals.
They're very aggressive. They're big. They have very sharp teeth.
And worst of all, they're smart. This particular troop surrounded
our camp and divided into two contingents. One created a ruckus at
one end of our camp, while the other took advantage of the diversion
to swarm over our kitchen tent and loot the contents. It was full of
Western-style food. The baboons completely wiped out our supply
of that, which actually turned out to be a good thing. We had to re-
sort then to using local food; since Ahmed and our guides were In-
dians, that meant basically Indian food with African ingredients, and
the guides turned out to be great cooks. We felt like we were living
large—not for the first nor the last time—and we ate pretty well.
From then on we took great care to guard our food closely.

Matthew and I frequently went on recreational safaris in Africa, in Tanzania and Kenya's great Serengeti plains, savanna land.
Here's a letter Matthew sent me, explaining the context of a photograph he took of me when I had just finished a long run. I was
drenched in sweat, looking thirty and the picture of perfect health
while holding a cup of joe.

Dear Rod,

*This photograph was taken in Kenya on our cut-rate safari
led by Ahmed the Guide. It reminded me of your idiotic 5K run
last year through that patch of jungle where a pride of lions was
known to be hunting [and in fact had killed a woman a week
earlier] along the Upper Zambezi River in Zimbabwe. It was
right after we returned from a six-day Upper Zambezi river*

trip in two-man kayaks, fearlessly dodging crocodiles as well as
hippos. That was also the day I polished off over a dozen steaks
in front of you at the Victoria Falls Hotel evening BBQ.

And you did charge a Cape buffalo on a run in Tanzania
during one of our DIY safaris. I was at the wheel of
Newsweek's Land Rover that morning, ready to scoop you
up if the Cape B looked remotely angry when you got close.
I remember you were waving a panga machete as you ran
down the dirt road in its direction. What we lacked in adult
supervision that trip we made up for in adventure.

It is great having photographer friends at such moments. What
I remember most from it was not the harrowing encounters with
hippos—which, in terms of human casualties, are by far the most
dangerous animals in Africa (with the exception of that most gratuitously violent of primates, man-unkind, as E. E. Cummings put
it—one of the few animals that routinely kills its own kind). Hippos are even more dangerous than lions, and all those crocs in the
Zambezi River. Crocs and hippos tended to gather in the large, still
pools that form in the river at the foot of each set of class III and
IV rapids. Matthew and I were both pretty good kayakers and were
able to maneuver away from the hippos and crocs safely after each
run. So that wasn't too worrisome.

What *was* worrisome happened one night on another safari trip
when we had pitched camp. A lion came strolling through the middle of our little encampment. It was a female—they're the ones
to worry about, the hunters. The males mostly sleep, help eat the
females' kills, and copulate. It's possible during mating season to
drive your vehicle right up to a pair of mating lions and see them in
action, up close and personal.

Mating lions engage in what humans would call rough sex. It
really looks like a fight to the death is going on when they copulate.

The growling, roaring, and biting seem so in earnest, it's amazing they don't actually draw blood—but they don't. One soon sees why the lion is called the king of beasts. The male quite often will have intercourse with one female multiple times an hour, and sometimes with several females multiple times in an afternoon, making a horrific noise every time he reaches completion. It's pretty unforgettable, especially up close. Fortunately these animals don't consider vehicles to be possible sources of prey. So if you're in a vehicle, even an open-bedded or open-backed one, you're pretty safe. I guess the lions have learned that they can't chew their way through sheet metal. Rhinos and Cape buffaloes have not, however, learned such a lesson and will quite readily charge and smash into motor vehicles several times their size.

Our guide on the riverine safari, Cecil, a former Rhodesian scout, barely shrugged at first when the female lion stepped into our midst. He had been among the pretty formidable characters who ran "Lurps," or long-range patrols, small teams of mostly white scouts who hunted down and killed "terrorists," as the white Rhodesians dubbed all of their opponents during Zimbabwe's war for independence from the white regime, in what was then Rhodesia. As in so many postcolonial conflicts, this truism held: *One man's terrorist is another man's freedom fighter.* A good corollary to that logical construct might run thus: *If your enemies are numerous, and all terrorists, you're probably on the wrong, or at least the losing, side.*

Cecil was also a font of homespun African aphorisms. One in particular has long stayed with me: "There are few problems in life that cannot be solved with either high explosives or duct tape; always keep a good supply of both."

When that lioness paraded through our riverside campground, we asked Cecil, who had a pistol strapped on his hip, why he didn't seem inclined to use its high explosives on her. He had instead picked up some pots and pans and began banging them, and fed more wood onto our campfire; his several Zimbabwean assistants did the same with whatever noisy things they could find, creating a hideous racket to pierce the stillness of the jungle night. They did this until the lion was startled or maybe confused enough to leave the camp, looking insouciantly back over her shoulder as she sauntered off. Cecil's reply to our question: "Are you crazy? I would never shoot an animal that beautiful. This gun is not for animals. It's for people."

Matthew and I put bedding on the roof of our Land Rover for the safety of our female companions. A couple of them took refuge from the scary night noises of the jungle—the low, throaty growling of our local pride on patrol, the high-pitched fire-alarm screaming of monkeys far more harmless than they sound—by retreating into the safety of the vehicle.

Matthew and I stayed up all night, nervously, obsessively feeding the campfire, which soon became a bonfire. Most creatures that can hurt you stay away from fire. Just outside the ring of light the flames cast, in the bushy margins, we could see the beady little eyes of numerous hyenas reflecting the firelight, as they watched in readiness. Campers in Africa are well warned that hyenas are quite capable of clamping their teeth into a foot sticking out the end of a sleeping bag and making off with a substantial chunk of flesh. So we slept with our boots on, as close to the fire as possible.

"BAGHDAD GARDEN BECOMES
GRAVEYARD, FULL OF GRIEVING"
New York Times
November 27, 2009

BAGHDAD, Iraq . . .

This garden, known as the Martyrs of Adhamiya since it became a cemetery in 2007, is so densely packed with graves that it is often difficult to walk between the rectangular capstones that cover each one (out of reverence, no one dares tread on top). Six months ago, the authorities counted 9,000 graves, but many more have been added since. Nearly all are victims of Iraqi-on-Iraqi violence of one sort or another: terroristic bombings, sectarian killings, political assassinations.

The air is scented with a profusion of burning joss sticks, stuck in the earth around the graves. Many are adorned, in the Iraqi way, with plastic flowers; often photographs of the deceased are propped up against the headstones.

Here no one seems to believe the war is over. "Even in a hundred years it won't get better," says Sabriya Fadhil Abbas, kneeling at the grave of her brother Ali, 39, killed by a car bomb in 2008, leaving a wife and seven children, the eldest 13. "They're still fighting in the government; no one trusts one another. How can it end?"

Unlike most of the graves, her brother's was covered with a corrugated roof on a simple metal framework. "To protect him from the sun and the rain," Ms. Abbas explains. At her feet was a bowl with Id pastries known as klecha; she offered them to well-wishers. Her mother will come later, she said; she can no longer walk, so her surviving sons will carry her from the mosque. A beggar woman comes by and scoops a handful of the klecha into the folds of her chador.

The family recently buried another member in the cemetery who was killed in the October bombing of the Ministry of Justice.

Alaa Adel, the best friend of Issam al-Obeidi, a local journalist, is here, killed by a sniper. "No Iraqi lives far away from all this," he says. Among those interred here is Khalid Hassan, a *New York Times* reporter and interpreter killed on his way to work in 2007.

People stand prayerfully before the graves, with both hands cupped before them, as if holding unseen weights.

CHAPTER 8

One Way to Be Born,
a Thousand Ways to Die

The first time I ever saw a dead person, early in my career abroad, I saw a hundred of them at one time, scattered over a Cambodian killing field in the Khao-i-Dang refugee camp. At the time this was the world's largest refugee camp, with hundreds of thousands of residents. Initially home to Cambodians fleeing the genocidal regime of the Khmer Rouge, the camp was later swollen with Khmer Rouge followers who were fleeing Vietnam's invasion of Cambodia, which would put an end to their regime, and then riven by factional infighting, motivated by greed not ideology, as gangs fought over the profits to be made from stealing international food aid. They were like a pack of hyenas fighting over the carcass of a half-decayed piece of game. That was what had populated that field I saw at the dawn of my career as a war correspondent with all those bodies. I have never expunged this image from my memory: all those bodies, men and women, gender often obscured by wounds and decomposition; a few children; each body, with its own buzzing canopy of flies, left in the grotesque position a violent death had imparted to it, many of them rapidly decomposing in the tropical heat. The gases released by that process caused their abdominal cavities to inflate like hideous balloons.

By 2007, I had seen many more such victims, in many other places. By then I was the chief foreign correspondent for *Newsweek*, and its Baghdad bureau chief in Iraq, one of six war zones where I've managed staffs of up to a hundred or more. By that time I had already covered wars in Central America, the former Yugoslavia, Somalia, Afghanistan—both when the Russians were getting eviscerated there and when the Americans had the delusion they could do better. I had also been in Iraq during Saddam Hussein's rule, to cover the Iran–Iraq War, and in Kuwait, for the Americans' First Gulf War.

In 2007, while I was working in Iraq, *Newsweek* assigned me an article about a US Army program called Combat Stress Teams. Groups of uniformed psychologists, mental health aids, and nurses were sent into the field in the midst of operations to find soldiers who exhibited signs of PTSD. The idea was to catch them early and get them the help and support they needed before they became even more traumatized. The photo desk at *Newsweek* assigned Gary Knight to shoot the story. Gary was a friend and colleague, and we had already worked in half a dozen war zones together during the previous decade.

We were near Tikrit, in central Iraq, interviewing the first sergeant in charge of one of the teams. This woman, like most first sergeants of any gender, was tough as tacks, with a no-nonsense, don't-mess-with-me attitude. Out of the blue she suggested that both Gary and I take the routine PTSD screening test they were giving to soldiers. What the hell, we said, and did so. As it turned out, my score indicated that I had moderate to severe PTSD. In for a penny, in for a pound. The army's protocol in cases like mine was to insist that the person get therapy with someone who knew how to treat PTSD—so I did.

Mandating PTSD screening, along with free, confidential psychotherapy, has now been widely adopted as a best practice by the whole raft of civilians who work in war zones, from contractors to journalists to workers in humanitarian organizations. Witnessing a suicide bombing can be a horrific experience—the violence and the blood, the arbitrary obliteration of lives, and the horrible vision of what high explosives can do to the human body—and the effects can linger for many years. In much the same way, some soldiers are haunted by their battlefield experiences for decades to come.

After this initial screening, it became obvious to me that as the bureau chief in Iraq, I needed to persuade management to require that everyone who had worked in war zones, whether as local staff, freelancers, photographers, reporters, or correspondents for any length of time, should undergo PTSD screening and an initial therapeutic assessment, with follow-up treatment if that was recommended. Confidentiality was key: no one would know who had undergone this process or what the outcome was. Even though the photographer was a longtime friend, I never asked Gary how he scored on his screening, and I never found out. I made no secret of mine and was referred for at least two months of weekly therapy sessions, making the process, in my case, public, to set a good example that would encourage others to do the same.

My therapist used a standard PTSD treatment, rapid eye movement desensitization and reprocessing, or EMDR. It helps the subject relive and face up to serious traumatic experiences. It is a way to recover from those experiences by vividly reexperiencing them in a controlled, safe, and supportive environment. As those experiences are relived and visualized, a remarkable reckoning takes place; they are no less real but somehow become much less traumatic and debilitating. What surprised both me and the therapist, however, was that by the conclusion of my sessions, it was clear that the root of my trauma was not witnessing the violence and carnage of war, but rather my childhood experience with my father; my PTSD had his fingerprints—and belt welts—all over it.

Curiously, that may be why working in war zones has never fazed me—except when I've witnessed the suffering of women and children. And perhaps this is why I've managed to do it for forty years, through nearly twenty-five conflicts, from Cambodia in 1979 to Syria in 2019. Unlike some of my colleagues—and certainly some soldiers I knew—I never got any kind of thrill from the violence and drama of war.

Me, I didn't miss it. Far from it. Often, I was terrified, as all sensible people should be when in the midst of the atrocities of war. Only stupid people aren't afraid; anybody with an ounce of sense or humanity is scared witless.

I didn't imagine in 1979, when I said goodbye to my family and headed off to Bangkok to open the Asia bureau of the *Philadelphia Inquirer*, that I would never truly come home to live in the United States again—not until a brain tumor, four decades later, forced my repatriation. The only exception was the year that my mother was dying of stage 4 cervical cancer; *Newsweek* let me work from Philly so I could help care for her. After I had covered Asia and then Central America for Gene Roberts, *Newsweek* lured me away in late 1994 to run their Beirut bureau in the midst of the Lebanese Civil War. This was the golden age for newsmagazines, all bulging expense accounts and a commitment to big, important stories. I stayed at *Newsweek* for the next twenty years, a period in news spanning the Contras in Nicaragua to the wars in Iraq and Afghanistan.

Then, in 2009, the *New York Times* hired me to be a foreign correspondent in their Baghdad bureau, then moved me to Kabul in 2011. By 2015, the *Times* made me international correspondent at large, and I succeeded Alissa Rubin as bureau chief in Kabul, one of the paper's biggest bureaus. Mostly, I settled in Iraq and Afghanistan, also taking a few detours into South Africa and Lebanon and Morocco. In Turkey my work led to my detention in Istanbul, and the country banned me for five years as a national security risk. I covered the Santa Claus tourist industry in Finland, the anti-Semites in Lithuania, and of course, India, when the local bureau chief wanted to take a vacation.

For all that time, from my youth well into my late middle age, I had faced down death, my own or others', in 150 different countries, most of them living through violent upheavals. I spent time in terrorist camps in the Middle East and wrote a cover story for *Newsweek* in 1986 titled "American Is Our Target," about the training of young men, efforts that were hiding in plain sight, which one could argue led directly to the attacks of 9/11.

But strangely, I never once thought that I would die in a war zone. Even when I was pinned down by hostile fire, saw people killed around me, and otherwise found myself in the approximate vicinity of something that could easily have killed me. I was convinced, somewhat superstitiously, that when I met my maker, it would be in a bathtub. Indeed, I've been wary of bathtubs almost my entire adult life. This fear is not entirely unfounded. In my twenties, I once slipped and fell while taking a shower in the bathtub. I hit my head hard against the tiled wall and was nearly knocked out—I felt so dizzy, I was unable to climb out of the bathtub safely. I just lay there until I realized my scalp was bleeding heavily. An odd sort of peace came over me, as I spun the narrative of the tragic end of the promising journalist, lying there and bleeding out, not discovered until the cleaner arrived later.

One of the dangers of being a foreign correspondent, or perhaps just an unintended consequence, is becoming an old bore, mired in past wars and spewing vivid but dated anecdotes. I don't want to be *that person*, and this book is about the very different combat zone in which I now find myself—it's not just about the previous ones. But as I look back, as I ponder mortality and the certainty that I now have more yesterdays than tomorrows, I can't help but reflect on some of my extraordinary near misses when I was young, physically strong, and confident of my invulnerability. And those near misses seemed to mark my various postings; they've become windows into slivers of time, albeit formative ones.

One of those events took place when I was in Thailand for the *Inquirer*. One night, a small group of colleagues and I sat playing gin rummy as we waited to be executed the next morning. We had torn pages from our notebooks and made a crude deck of cards, but the soldiers who were guarding us indignantly confiscated them, pronouncing card games illegal. "Oh, but extrajudicial killings are OK, is that it?" I asked, in my bad but serviceable Thai. "*Hubpak*," one of the soldiers said—which, in rough translation, means "Shut the fuck up."

This was in 1980, when the army from Vietnam had invaded Cambodia and was destroying the Hun Sen and Khmer Rouge regime. The enormous Khao-i-Dang refugee camp had been hastily created in Thailand for Cambodians fleeing after the fall of the Khmer Rouge. Hundreds of thousands gathered there. A group of Thai soldiers had taken me and a few fellow journalists captive because they were deeply angered that we had seen them on the Cambodian side of the Thai border—where they were forbidden to go. I had found that Thai soldiers were also directing the Cambodian guerrilla forces that were fighting the Vietnamese—they did not appreciate my knowing this fact, much less reporting it for the *Inquirer*. I can't imagine they had any concept of what the esteemed *Philadelphia Inquirer* really was, but they did know that we were reporters and therefore enemies. They arrested us and declared they would execute us in the morning.

When faced with an unpleasant but unavoidable circumstance, I am blessed with a helpful reflex: I fall asleep. For instance, I'm absolutely terrified of landing on aircraft carriers. During the First

Gulf War, we journalists often flew in a transport plane out to an aircraft carrier, where we stayed for weeks at a time, embedded with the sailors and aviators. Landing a plane on a carrier generally requires deploying a tail hook that must catch a three-inch-thick steel cable lifted across the deck runway during the plane's approach, at over a hundred miles an hour. When the fast-moving plane hits the deck, it is hooked to a dead stop in a couple of seconds. When I flew on one of those planes, the only way I could face that sudden landing was to flip my sleep switch and go dead asleep, waking up once we had slammed to the deck and were hooked to the stop. Upon opening my eyes, I was shocked awake and delighted to be alive. This delight in being alive has become more frequent these days. A terminal illness will do that for you.

On the eve of our promised execution, my friends were incredulous, not to mention mildly outraged, when I zoned out. "Your last night alive, and you're going to spend it sleeping?" one fellow journalist asked. "Yes," I replied, "and get a good rest so that first thing in the morning I can jump that fence and run like hell into the jungle." The soldiers had no idea what we were talking about, but they didn't like the sound of it. "*Hubpak*," they repeated. When I woke up, I saw a Red Cross delegation. Throughout the world, ICRC representatives visit detention places of all sorts. Once they saw us and took our names, we knew that we would be safe. When news of our imprisonment leaked out, an international furor ensued. Gene Roberts leaned on Richard Holbrooke, then the US assistant secretary of state. Though Holbrooke personally hated my guts, he leaned on our Thai allies to release us, knowing that complying might well have negative consequences for them.

I learned an important lesson during those border skirmishes. I was internally still the eighteen-year-old tough guy from Philly, and like so many young men, I had not realized that I might be mortal. That attitude ended the day I foolishly went up to the front line during one of those pointless factional skirmishes. That was the time, mentioned earlier, when a fighter was head-shot, and his distraught comrades forced me at gunpoint to take him to the hospital in my Avis rental car. That victim and I had been standing shoulder to shoulder, listening to bullets whiz over our heads. The bullet that hit him could just as easily have killed me. After that terrifying realization, I was shaking for days. I never again allowed myself anywhere near the front line in a gun battle.

I left Thailand when my four-year tour was up, but I wanted to remain a foreign correspondent. I persuaded Gene to let me settle in San Salvador and dive into the wars in Central America—where death squads, those groups of armed killers, many of them former policemen from the regime of the previous dictator of Nicaragua, Anastasio Somoza, would regularly assassinate political opponents. Journalists would go out every morning, cruising the streets to look for bodies, and we were seldom disappointed. Sometimes the squads would save us the trouble, dumping the bodies of victims in the parking lot of the El Camino Real Hotel. On one occasion these killers, who frequently filled our hotel letter boxes with death threats, named all the journalists based there and gave us each a number, saying that was our position on the list of those to be killed. (I was a little disappointed to be assigned a high number.) Once, they dropped a body off in the parking lot of the hotel, with a press release pinned to the victim's shirt.

The most notorious attacks came in 1980, at the cathedral in San Salvador, when an enormous crowd of anti-government protesters gathered. Bombs were set off in the crowd while gunmen fired wildly into it; dozens more were killed in the terrified stampedes the attack set off. Inside the church, while Archbishop Oscar Romero was saying mass, he was assassinated by a member of a death squad, a UN inquiry later concluded.

I divided my time between El Salvador and Nicaragua. A civil war had been raging since 1980 in El Salvador, and now the Reagan administration was pouring massive military assistance into the country. In Nicaragua, a Communist-leaning government was being attacked by US-supported Contras. During the Reagan administration, Central America was the dominant foreign story of the day. It's hard to imagine it now, but the El Camino Real Hotel in San Salvador, a sleepy capital city of a tiny country, hosted twenty-five news bureaus in its rooms, including one for the *Philadelphia Inquirer*.

Over the years, in many parts of the world, I have witnessed, or even assisted, when injured colleagues were medevacked out of a war zone. The first such experience was in Nicaragua, where the Sandinistas were firmly in control, which alarmed the Americans because the Sandinistas had an avidly anti-American, anti-Western socialist outlook. Eden Pastore, one of the original Sandinista leaders, had turned against the group when their socialist leanings became apparent; he formed a breakaway faction of Sandinista fighters who came to be called the Contras. They were very quickly embraced by the Reagan administration and the American military; their leaders considered the Sandinistas terrorists. The United States lavishly financed the Contras and Eden Pastore as they carried out their breakaway war.

In May 1984, Pastore announced a press conference at his camp in Northern Nicaragua, close to the Costa Rican border. It was such an obvious target, I had little doubt that the Sandinistas would attack it. Always willing to play the coward when necessary, I didn't go. I decided to do what we called "coverback"—talking to people who were there and piecing together what had happened after the event. Susan Morgan, a forty-year-old part-time correspondent for *Newsweek*, had covered this war for a long time and was steeped in the cause of the Sandinistas. She saw the press conference as a great opportunity, and against the advice of her editors, she wanted to go.

They weren't interested in the story and didn't think it was worth the bother, but she went anyway, as did a phony journalist carrying a bomb.

The explosive was planted next to Pastore and set off with a cell phone, killing twelve of those present, badly wounding Eden Pastore, and mangling Susan Morgan.

Susan, her face battered, her eyes injured, her arms and legs fractured, was taken by Pastore's people to a jungle hospital of dubious reputation. She was part of a lefty, pro-Sandinista community based in Costa Rica and Central America. Her friends, extremely politically correct, felt it would be an odious form of cultural imperialism to suggest that this hospital, in middle-of-nowhere Costa Rica, was anything less than a suitable place for her to be treated.

This, of course, was nonsense. The place was a dump, the floors filthy, an obvious unhygienic mess, staffed by people who seemed at best marginally competent. They could not take care of someone in Susan's state. Having arrived in Northern Nicaragua after the bombing, I called *Newsweek* and explained that she was in bad shape in a bad hospital, and encouraged the staff to medevac her, which they immediately agreed to and asked me to arrange. It was then I learned that my theoretically-no-limit American Express card truly had no limit. I used it to book a $24,000 jet ambulance, with a nurse and a doctor aboard, to fly to a jungle landing strip in Costa Rica, pick up Susan, and depart for Gainesville, Florida, where Susan would get proper care at the medical school of the University of Florida, the nearest level 1 trauma center.

I got on board with her and the medical team, and when we arrived in Gainesville, Susan's boyfriend appeared. He seemed to be very troubled by how serious her injuries were, and shockingly, he couldn't bring himself to hold her hand before she was wheeled away to surgery. So I held her hand, even though I scarcely knew her. In the end she had something like ten major operations before she was stabilized and out of danger.

I was still at the *Inquirer* when all this happened. The experience with Susan served as a kind of introduction to the foreign desk at *Newsweek*. There were so many correspondents in Central America at the time that I am not sure I stood out as particularly notable. But when the *Newsweek* staff saw how I handled Susan's situation, how quickly and effectively I organized her evacuation, as the editor Maynard Parker later told me, they opened a file on me as a potential recruit. They reached out, and after a few meetings, they decided to hire me later that year, nearly doubling my salary and offering me all the glories that newsmagazines had to offer at the time: a generous expense account, incredible opportunities to travel, the assurance that there would be very few constraints on me when there was a story I wanted to cover.

After more than ten years of an incredibly rich experience in journalism, from covering cops and courts and popes to amazing adventures all over the world, I felt that the professional home I had with the *Inquirer*—and indeed it was my hometown paper—was like nothing I would ever again enjoy. Sure, I would have great experiences over the next nearly four decades of my career, but there was something about the growth that took place for me there, from a kid, really, with lots of ambition and talent to a seasoned foreign correspondent. No place could have trained me for the rest of my life the way that paper under Gene Roberts did.

Gene Roberts gave his correspondents total freedom as writers, more than any other paper then or since, and there was no story he wouldn't let us do. Gene faced pressure from the rest of the Knight Ridder chain over the heavy costs of his new foreign bureaus, but his commitment to spending the money that was needed for great journalism soon produced eight Pulitzers for the *Inquirer* in a year—

more than any other regional paper since World War II, aside from the powerhouses of the *New York Times* and *Washington Post*. One year we won four Pulitzers. During my time with Gene, I garnered two Polk Awards among many other prizes, and was a Pulitzer finalist for international reporting. Gene cannily created an entire department, staffed by several of his most talented lieutenants, that was dedicated to entering and winning award competitions.

So, it was with no small measure of guilt that I let *Newsweek* recruit me for its Beirut bureau at the height of the civil war there. Gene and many other colleagues tried to talk me out of taking the job, but I wanted a more powerful forum, one that played on a world stage, which was something the *Inquirer*, no matter how good, no matter how prizewinning, could never do.

In early 1985 I headed over to Beirut, to cover a very different kind of conflict. I had war-zone experience, and *Newsweek* needed that because there was a major civil war going on in Beirut, involving the Palestinians as well as factions of the Lebanese. When I arrived, the city was shelling itself. People were planting bombs or cars full of explosives all over the place, which would blow up and, in some cases, kill half the people in the neighborhood. There was a wave of kidnappings and assassinations of westerners by Hezbollah and Islamic Jihad, and active warfare went on in the southern suburbs and outskirts of the city.

Yet Beirut was an enchanting city. In the spring and late summer, when you could see snow on Mount Lebanon in the mountains, the *met'n*, as they call it, to the east and south of the city, it was also warm enough to go swimming. The city has been destroyed so many times and been through so much conflict that the Beirut Lebanese have become experts at rebuilding. Seemingly the minute a building was smashed by shelling or bombs, workmen appeared to bring it all back to life. There was energy there, born of resilience and life on the edge, when death and the obliteration of all that you have taken for granted seem imminent. In many ways, Beirut was a city in a perpetual state of living its Second Life.

I moved into a small apartment building on the Corniche owned by a guy named Walid, who would sit in his front hallway with a rocket-propelled grenade launcher between the legs of his chair. He had lined up a point-blank shot for unwelcome visitors, ensuring they never came through again. Another denizen of the building was Robert Fisk, a British journalist who worked for the once venerable British paper the *Independent*. Fisk was popular in Britain and among college audiences in the United States, where he supplemented his living by giving speeches denouncing US foreign policy and nearly everything else about the country—some of his criticisms were based in fact, but many were not. Among colleagues who worked with him in the field, Fisk had a reputation as a fabulist. His book, *Pity the Nation*, became the go-to volume on Lebanon's war, despite being full of falsehoods and rank inventions. When I moved into the same building, it seemed to trigger Fisk's most paranoid anti-American fantasies.

Shortly before I arrived, William Buckley, the CIA station chief in Beirut since 1983, was kidnapped while leaving his apartment. Buckley's abduction set in motion the series of events that, improbably, would lead me back to Central America. Colonel Oliver North drafted a national security directive on getting hostages released from Iran—hostage taking was big business in the Middle East at the time. It was Reagan's second term, and the plan was to secretly break the arms embargo to Iran by selling them weapons, then using the funds from those sales to support the Contras in Nicaragua—whose support had been curtailed by Congress. When the arms shipments began, they were justified as a way to free Buckley and six other hostages that Hezbollah had seized in Lebanon. It did no good. Buckley was tortured and assassinated by Imad Fayez Mughniyeh, one of Hezbollah's ranking leaders and a notorious terrorist.

This became known as the Iran-Contra affair, a major scandal of the Reagan administration. I had only a small point of intersection with Buckley: Fisk noted the coincidence of my arrival in Beirut close to the time when Buckley was kidnapped, and he concocted the insane theory that I had been assigned the job as the new CIA station chief. This idea was not just demented but also a falsehood that made things extremely dangerous for me.

Living in Beirut at the time had the quality of a Graham Greene novel, a dangerous but beautiful backdrop populated by many people who were working various angles. My driver, Mehdi, was solicitous of my safety and insisted that I hire a bodyguard. It turned out that the bodyguard he had in mind was his brother, Ali. Those were dramatic days in Beirut, and it was not uncommon for a mortar shell to hit my building. I hired Ali as my bodyguard, albeit with a certain reluctance; the world of official bodyguards was new territory for me, and as a general rule, hiring an employee's relative is never a good idea.

We all worked in a fully functioning bureau downtown that was occupied by *Newsweek* and Worldwide Television News—a British company that no longer exists. Our two organizations shared the facility and split the costs. The bureau was run by a Palestinian fellow named Abdul Majid who had worked for quite a long time for WTN. Abdul billed both *Newsweek* and WTN for the same expenses, which meant that the rent and utility bills were all paid twice, with Abdul pocketing the surplus. Then he began demanding kickbacks from staff—fixers, drivers, translators—at 20 percent of their pay. Some of them rebelled, and a WTN employee decided to report this transgression to London. Not long after, as that employee was walking down Hamra Street, a sniper put a bullet in his head. We suspected an arranged assassination because this guy had reported Abdul's grift. Hamra then was Druze turf, and the Druze made sure to keep the peace, so a sniper killing was unexpected and immediately aroused suspicions.

To some extent, in a war zone you expected a certain amount of petty theft from your employees, particularly an operator like Abdul, who was good at getting things done, such as getting permits to cross the Green Line in Beirut. Naturally, he would deploy the skills that made him adept at these tasks in his internal work at the bureau. He was very useful; he was also, it turned out, very dangerous.

Following the assassination, WTN decided to close its part of the bureau, thereby cutting Abdul's income in half and leaving me and *Newsweek* holding the bag. A few days later, Terry Anderson, the AP bureau chief, was kidnapped after a game of tennis. He ended up being held prisoner by Islamic Jihad for almost seven years. A number of other Western hostages were taken as well, including a professor from the American University of Beirut and a couple of other journalists from Britain. All of them remained prisoners for many years. Terry Waite, an Anglican churchman and a peace envoy, showed up to try to work out a deal that would get the hostages released, but Islamic Jihad immediately took him hostage as well, holding him for more than four years.

The same day that Terry Anderson was taken, I left the *Newsweek* bureau on Hamra Street downtown and said goodbye to Abdul and our news assistant, Sana Issa. "Take care out there," Abdul said as I left. "It's dangerous these days." I hadn't told him I now had a bodyguard. I stepped out of the building onto Hamra Street and was immediately surrounded by five guys showing me the pistols held in their waistbands. My bodyguard, Ali, courageously faced them all down with his own 9mm automatic pistol. "Just run," Ali whispered to me, which I did, straight back to the bureau. This sounds impossibly courageous, but Ali was well aware that since these gunmen were Shiites and we were on Druze turf, any gunplay on their part would breach the uneasy truce then in place among Beirut's many warring factions. When I got back up to the bureau, opened the door, and stepped in, I saw the look of shock on Abdul's face. I felt sure that he had set me up and had expected never to see me again.

Clearly Abdul had to go. I conferred with *Newsweek*'s chief of correspondents, Bob Rivard, whom I had known in Central America. We decided to invite Abdul on a vacation to Paris as a reward for his splendid service to *Newsweek*. Abdul was sufficiently vain to fall for it. As he flew to Paris, I removed his name from our bank accounts, changed the bureau locks, and reset the combination on the safe. Rivard met him at our bureau in Paris and confronted him with the evidence that we had compiled about how much money he had stolen, and how he had compromised the safety of our staff. Naturally, Abdul smoothly blamed me, saying that I had ordered him to do all the skimming and double billing. Indeed, he said, I had pocketed all the proceeds myself. Rivard knew that this was utter bullshit, and he ended the conversation by bodily pushing Abdul out the door of the Paris bureau and firing him.

That ended our relationship with Abdul Majid. But not entirely. Once he returned to Beirut, he began repeating Robert Fisk's lie that I was the new CIA station chief.

Fisk's vile rumor has popped up in odd places. Once I ran into a German reporter at the bar of the Nile Hilton in Cairo, and he began telling me about a journalist named "Rod Nordland," whom he claimed to know quite well.

"Do tell," I said, fascinated to hear more about this guy.

It was well known, he said, that Nordland had been sent to Beirut as the CIA station chief to replace William Buckley after he was kidnapped, with his job as *Newsweek* bureau chief as his cover. I asked him where he got this information, and he replied that it came from one of the best-informed journalists in Beirut, Robert Fisk. Then, to further underscore Fisk's credibility, he said that Fisk was also Nordland's neighbor in the Hamra section of Beirut. That at least was true; our apartments were on different floors of Walid's well-guarded building on the Corniche.

"So do you actually know this guy Nordland?" I asked.

"Of course I do," he replied.

"That's odd," I said, "because I am Rod Nordland, you asshole." I think my anger alone was enough to make him physically retreat, uttering some lame apology. As soon as I returned to Beirut, I confronted Fisk, who denied ever having said this. He allowed that he might have mentioned the odd coincidence that my arrival had occurred within a few months of Buckley's kidnapping. I was furious and pointed out the obvious fact that even this kind of talk could get me killed. I demanded an apology and told him to correct the record with everyone he had shared his stupid theory with. Fisk left the bar mumbling "Sorry," and that's the last we spoke for several years. When he was arrested in Diyarbakir by Turkish police and appealed to me to get the American embassy to help him, I did so. I couldn't stay in Beirut any longer, however, so I continued to cover the Lebanese conflict from Cyprus.

Then, in 1987, I returned to Central America, to a story that refused to go away. The Contras of Nicaragua were a different paramilitary entity altogether, more of an organized force backed by US government military equipment and funding and coordinated by the CIA and its paramilitary operatives in Northern Nicaraguan and Honduran border areas. In the United States, the story of Colonel Oliver North and others in the Reagan administration and their bizarre plans to liberate the country from the yoke of Communism was beginning to be revealed. Many of us who worked in Central America doubted the narrative that the Contras were beloved by their countrymen, but only a few journalists were allowed to get close to the paramilitary group long enough to see.

After months of negotiation in Washington with various high-ranking officials involved with supporting them, the Contras agreed to my request, as a *Newsweek* reporter, to accompany them. (I'm still amazed that they did.) They said that the photographer Bill Gentile and I could go with them for a month. So we set out with a unit of

120 Contras under a *comandante* named Attila and went into the field. It turned out to be the most physically grueling month of my life. Not all of the Contras were thrilled to have us traveling with them. They were constantly running short on food and provisions, and not only were we two more mouths to feed, but we also slowed their progress as they played a game of cat-and-mouse with the Sandinista army. In reality, we spent most of our time either fleeing or hiding from the Sandinistas. As soon as it was dark, we would burrow into the underbrush at the edge of the jungle and literally bury ourselves in piles of weeds and brambles so that we would be completely invisible from the air. The Sandinistas had Soviet-made helicopters, which we did our best to evade.

In the mornings, we would wake up before dawn and crawl out of our holes to hear from the scouts how close the Sandinista column was. Usually they were a mile away—that was the distance from which their snipers could hit us. Our group's interaction with the Nicaraguan public made them no friends. Sometimes we wouldn't see the Sandinistas for a whole day, or even two days if we got a good lead on them, and so we spent that time visiting local small farmers and asking them for "donations" of food and provisions, which often turned out to mean stripping their farms of nearly everything they had. Their public relations machine in Washington continued to depict them as winning hearts and minds throughout Nicaragua. The reality was quite the reverse.

We journalists were always scared and usually hungry because the Contras did not care much about feeding us when supplies got tight. Camping and trekking in the mountains of Northern Nicaragua were also physically grueling. I learned a lot of things on that march, such as how to go down a very steep slope safely while carrying a heavy pack, and also how to carefully decide which trees to use to help keep your balance or support you while ascending.

Once we came to the hut of a campesino named Obediente. The

Contras had taken his last chicken, any eggs they could find, his beans and his rice, and a burlap sack of coffee beans, which I presumed was his only cash crop. He was one of the lucky ones, though; often the Contras kidnapped peasants to make them walk point in the column, in case of ambush or mines on the path. Obediente and his entire family suffered from mountain leprosy and were a two or three days' walk from the nearest government clinic. It felt like all we were doing was ravaging the countryside and making enemies for the Contras and, if anything, friends for the Sandinistas. One of those farmers who donated so much to them later confided this in private: "During the Sandinista time, we were poor, but we had enough. Now they leave us with nothing." As we left Obediente's farm, Comandante Attila said, "You saw how much they loved us, didn't you?"

My story in *Newsweek*—which ran on the cover and was titled "Inside the Contra War: Why They're Not Winning"—was a savage excoriation of the whole Contra operation and had a major impact on the national discourse about American aid to anti-Sandinista forces. Bill Gentile and I were attacked as Sandinista plants, but the story really was one of those rare occasions when the journalist gets to have a major impact on policy and the course of events. The story was widely cited as proof that our support of the Contras was a losing cause and became Exhibit A during the Iran-Contra scandal. To some extent, our work helped bring to an end Colonel Oliver North's dreams of covert American-supported wars against leftists in Nicaragua and El Salvador, Guatemala, and Colombia.

Every year it seemed as if there was another war. As the civil war in Lebanon was dying out, the First Gulf War in Iraq exploded, and I got more acquainted with that country, setting up *Newsweek*'s bureau in Baghdad. Then came the civil war in Yugoslavia in 1992, a hideous, nearly decade-long conflict that was the result of the ethnically heterogeneous country breaking up after Communism had somehow managed to keep it intact for over forty years. The Bosnian War lasted from 1992 until 1995, and then the Kosovo War exploded in 1998. And oh yes, the Russian occupation of Afghanistan, which offered me my first introduction to that godforsaken country when it was a battlefield.

I covered them all. I carried my backpack with my knife and water-purifying tablets, my notebooks and my satellite telephone, a change of clothes, and a Kevlar blanket, with its astonishing ability to keep you warm. I knew how to set up bureaus and find the best fixers and translators and bodyguards when necessary. I became the expert at negotiating with landlords in war-ravaged cities, and I always kept my eyes open for stories about children and women— casualties of men's immoral wars who were too easy to ignore.

I will write about Iraq and Afghanistan in a subsequent chapter, but as I reflect on my work in the 1980s and 90s, I am reminded of an observation by the Czech novelist Milan Kundera about a different period of time: "The bloody massacre in Bangladesh quickly covered over the memory of the Russian invasion of Czechoslovakia, the assassination of Allende drowned out the groans of Bangladesh, the war in the Sinai Desert made people forget Allende, the Cambodian massacre made people forget Sinai, and so on and so forth until ultimately everyone lets everything be forgotten."

Just insert different place-names; it's still the same, ad infinitum. I felt it was my job as a reporter to try to make sure that people didn't let everything be forgotten.

Except, of course, they did. How else to explain why it keeps happening.

KABUL, Afghanistan—The driver of a car that was stopped in the middle of the road, blocking traffic, was shocked when a passing motorist rolled down the window and shouted at him, "Dirty donkey."

He was even more surprised when he looked up to see that the insult came from a woman. A woman driving a car. A woman driving a car without wearing the obligatory hijab.

That was Laila Haidari, who runs a popular café in Kabul that allows men and women to dine together, whether married or not, with or without a head scarf, and uses the profits to fund a rehabilitation clinic for drug addicts.

Nearly everyone addresses Ms. Haidari, 39, as "Nana," or "Mom," and her supporters describe her as the "mother of a thousand children," after the number of Afghan addicts she has reportedly saved. . . .

Her nearly always crowded restaurant, on the banks of the sewage-drenched Kabul River, is named after a 15th-century warrior princess from Herat who helped rule a vast kingdom, a rare example of female power from that time.

Ms. Haidari is as unusual in her own age. . . .

"This is not just a restaurant," said one of the diners at Taj Begum, Ilyas Yourish, 24, a filmmaker. "It's a social center, a place to organize, and we all know she takes the money and puts it into the treatment center. Laila is the most powerful woman around here." . . .

Ms. Haidari's three children, now aged 16 to 21, have fled to Germany from Iran, and while she has not been able to visit them, she is in touch by WhatsApp.

Her work is for them, she said.

"I should have something to tell my own children and my grandchildren, when they ask, 'What did you do when the Taliban came?'"

CHAPTER 9

Searching for the Perfect Woman

There's a line that I've often thought characterizes my serious relationships: "I've spent my whole life searching for the perfect woman, but when I found her, she was still looking for the perfect man."

Somewhere between Lebanon and Bosnia I met Sheila. In the end, our relationship didn't work out any better than the many that came before. But we did find time to make three children together. And I managed to be home for the birth of each one, a feat that few war correspondents can claim to equal. We don't get days off in the foreign correspondent business, especially when covering wars. Most of these choices could have cost me my job. The chief of correspondents at *Newsweek* tried to fire me because I abandoned my post in Bosnia on the eve of the 1995 US intervention to be with Sheila for the birth of our second child, Johanna. In the end the late Maynard Parker, then the executive editor of *Newsweek*, intervened to protect me. Maynard was a terrific editor, especially in a crisis; he was famous for the expression he used when one arose: "Let's scramble the jets." I was always delighted to answer this summons. I was the guy who always had a visa ready, in one or another of the three or more passports I routinely carried, for wherever I might be summoned to go.

Sheila and I first crossed paths in Bahrain, where we both were attending a hash, a uniquely British cross-country running race popular all over the world. An informal international organization known as the Hash House Harriers conceived it. The pack of runners (the "hounds") follow a trail laid out in chalk by one of the harriers (the "hare"), and as they proceed, the contestants find that some of the trails lead nowhere, so when they find the true trail, they all yell "on" and resume chasing down the hare. There are water stations along the route. Except occasionally you would be handed a glass full of pure gin instead. Our hash event was held at seven or eight in the evening, but it being Bahrain, the temperature was still a toasty 120 degrees Fahrenheit.

The run ends with everyone gathering for what is poetically called the "Down Downs," a bizarre ritual reminiscent of a frat party. The name refers to downing drinks, and the hash's "grand master" presides over this. He commands participants to drink pints of beer as a penalty for any of several real or invented transgressions, such as allegedly taking a shortcut, wearing a new pair of sneakers, or sporting a T-shirt with a stupid slogan on it. The Down Downs typically takes place around a row of blocks of ice at the finish line—no easy feat to arrange when the temperature is soaring way over 100 degrees Fahrenheit. Then the transgressors, in addition to being penalized by quaffing beers, are required to pull their trousers down and sit bare-bottom on the blocks of ice. Just why this is, no one seems to know. Out of a twisted sense of chivalry, perhaps, only the men are thus penalized. The practical effect that night in Bahrain: my future wife had the dubious pleasure of seeing my bare ass before most any other part of me.

This event could have been just another debauched entertainment for expats (the hash's slogan: "a drinking club with a running problem"), but among them I saw a young Englishwoman—blond, beautiful, with an intelligent face. She was apparently unaccompanied, so during one of the breaks we started chatting. We got on splen-didly. I found that she was from a working-class family in England, and so she too understood the experience of growing up with no sense of security about what life might have in store. I learned she loved travel and hated dogs—rare in both our respective societies—and that alone might have been enough for me to be smitten. But then she also mentioned she loved playing squash. It seemed only natural that one of our next meetings would be at a squash court, and it marked the first of many times when she would clobber me. I was never a great squash player, as much as I loved the game. When my son, Jake, years later took up club play seriously—when we were living in Italy at one point, he was the fourth-ranked player in his age group in the country—it was a rare game when I could score more than one point against him. Sheila discouraged our playing together, describing it, correctly, alas, as "a waste of his court time."

And so, we began seeing each other, on and off, in Britain and Bahrain, or Ecuador, where she was then living, and the relation-ship deepened. I had turned forty a couple of years before and had watched all my siblings have children, feeling a bit of a pang, per-haps my male version of the biological clock. After so many years making homes wherever I happened to be deployed, I rather longed for a more permanent one, with a wife and a couple of kids. War correspondents tend to be cowboys, adventurers with a charming sense of detachment (so we think), and I surely was one. But I was also an idealist who wanted to give Sheila, and later my children, the security my own family had never had.

After Sheila and I met, and then married in 1991, when I was forty-two-years old, she began to accompany me on my various trips—which meant going to war zones. I felt it was important to "demythologize" war reporting, so she could see that it usually wasn't so dangerous for us war correspondents. I wanted her to see how all sides, even guerrillas, took care to protect us, at least until the days when extremist groups like Al Qaeda, and especially ISIS, threw out all the rules, and journalists—especially American ones— became highly sought after as targets and hostages (by the early 2000s, the reputed jihadi bounty for the capture of an American journalist was $2 million). But the early 1990s were more innocent days, when all sides, even guerrilla outfits, had a vested interest in keeping the press safe. So, if you proceeded with caution, diligence, and experience, the job could be done safely.

The best reporting was not done on the front lines but rather far behind them, at hospitals and command posts, where it was possible to safely talk to protagonists. I preached to my colleagues the virtues of cowardice. Anyone who wasn't scared to death amid high explosives and high-velocity projectiles was just a damn fool. Front lines were places for fools and combatants, and occasionally for some very brave photographers with little regard for their own lives. Over the years, I had figured out how to cover the hot spots without unduly jeopardizing myself. Before Sheila and I started a family, the whole world in which I lived needed to be seen with her own eyes, so that when she was home, she could be reassured of my well-being based on her own personal experience.

She was also able to reassure the children, who on occasion were made aware that their dad had a potentially dangerous job. When I first went to Baghdad and the kids were at a primary school in Beirut, where I was posted with the family for a couple years between its wars, the other children sometimes taunted ours: "Your dad's going to get killed in Baghdad." After Beirut came Rome, a place I had become fond of during my first overseas assignment, covering the deaths of the popes Paul VI and John Paul I in 1978 and then the election of pope John Paul II. Sheila and I set up housekeeping on the Via Appia Antica, the famous ancient Roman highway that cuts straight as an arrow across the middle of Italy, from Rome to Brindisi, down near the heel of the Italian boot, on the Adriatic

Sea. Our home was a small sylvan villa that previously had been the temporary home of Elizabeth Taylor during the making of a film in nearby Cinecittà, Italy's Hollywood.

In those days, satellite phones were cumbersome and expensive, about $10,000 each, compared to maybe $1,000 today. The models available in the early 1990s took up two heavy suitcases and were rather difficult to set up and operate. In many war zones, all the journalists used AP and other wire services' satellite phones to get in touch with their desks and families, but this came at an exorbitant cost, often as much as $100 a minute.

I hit on the idea of buying a satellite phone ourselves and then setting up shop to sell time on it at fair prices. Sheila had already learned how to operate the full-sized satellite phone that I was traveling with, so she had a head start. She basically set up a telephone office, charging a reasonable rate of about twenty dollars a minute, a modest markup on the rates the satellite telephone providers were charging us. I figured this approach would quickly pay off the cost of the machine. The service we offered was inexpensive enough to attract many clients. Eventually, Sheila came to be one of the most popular people in the war zones we visited, particularly in Kurdistan and northern Iraq.

The following year we bought our first house, in a London suburb called Cobham, halfway between Heathrow and Gatwick airports. This was a key location, since I had become a kind of fireman for *Newsweek* by then, covering conflicts from Asia to Africa and especially the Middle East. Sheila and I particularly liked working together in Kurdistan, along the Turkish border in a place called Diyarbakir, where we had a suite of rooms in the Diyarbakir Caravanserai, one of those historical inns on what was once the Silk Road. This one was some eight hundred years old and made of stone. It was the place where caravans would stop so the wranglers could sleep indoors, and rest and feed their camels and horses. For a time, the Diyarbakir Caravanserai became my informal base for covering the Kurds during the American intervention and the imposition of the no-fly zone over northern Iraq. I came to sympathize strongly with the Turkish Kurds—I especially appreciated their policy of taking the wages of abusive husbands and giving their wives the money. That really touched me where I lived; among his many abuses, my father had never paid my mother a dime of the court-ordered child support for us six kids. My attitude toward the Kurds led the Turkish government to ban me from the country as a national security risk.

It was the second country to ban me. The first, hilariously, was Mexico, which had declared me persona non grata after a 1983 *Newsweek* cover story I wrote was published. Among other things, it called the country one of the world's most dangerous places for tourists, after a string of high-profile murders of American tourists, some committed by *federales*, the Mexican national police force. I also noted that the country's capital, Mexico City, was becoming uninhabitable due to unprecedented levels of air pollution.

The story also predicted (correctly) that, thanks mostly to top-to-bottom corruption among officials, drug cartels were on their way to taking over the country, as they earlier had in Colombia.

In practice that ban was unenforceable; the US-Mexican border was wide open southbound, and I have visited Mexico many times since I was pronounced P.N.G.

Soon our children appeared. Lorine was born in 1992, at the beginning of the Bosnia War, and Johanna was born in 1995, while that conflict continued to grind on, and NATO and the United States finally put their soldiers where their mouths were and intervened militarily. Jake was born in 1998, the year Osama bin Laden and Al Qaeda announced themselves to Americans with the embassy bombing in Nairobi. At the time, long before Iraq was invaded by the Americans, it was a thorny foreign affairs issue, as Saddam took to using poison gas against his enemies, the Iranians and Kurds. My role as the children's provider was a source of profound satisfaction to me. But to give them a grounded life, I had to put my own at risk, roaming the world. And the truth is, I loved both the roaming and the risk. Sheila often described herself as a single mother with three children, which to a degree was true, although I was never really out of touch.

Once when the kids were little, Sheila had a migraine attack of such severity, she couldn't even dial a telephone; such attacks sometimes lasted a week for her. With little children to care for, she might not be able to call for help when she needed it. It was a real emergency. At the time we didn't have an au pair or nanny in residence, so she was alone. I was in a remote part of Bosnia then, days away from Rome, so I arranged for a friend of hers to fly in from Madrid for a week. The friend couldn't afford the trip, so I persuaded her that I could fly her in using only air miles (which wasn't true, as she suspected), but the important thing was that Sheila and the kids wouldn't be alone during one of those awful attacks. I have a great deal of empathy for migraine sufferers—most of the women I've known well have been among them. Migraines are so debilitating, and they strike usually without warning, often to a crippling degree; oddly, it's almost always women who are afflicted. Many migraineurs, as chronic sufferers are termed, experience what they describe as auras before an attack, a mental premonition hard to describe. I imagine they are like the auras I used to experience prior to seizures, in the days before my neurologists found the right combination of anti-seizure meds and pretty much eliminated them—my last confirmed seizure was on April 15, 2021. (I know this because I was on the phone with one of my neurologists when it struck, and he detected it through my slurred speech.)

Our children grew up as citizens of the world, with a passion for travel. I am never sure which countries they are all in at any given time. Johanna made friends at each hotel pool, and because she is so warm and outgoing, everywhere she went, she drew people to her like a human magnet. Jake would graduate magna cum laude with a bachelor's degree in foreign affairs, but instead of following Dad into a foreign affairs career, he invented a career all his own as an e-sports journalist, covering both the business and the sport of that fast-growing pursuit. He managed to turn this into a full-time job, with benefits, for a leading e-sports website. After all those years that my ex-wife and I worried about him spending long hours video-gaming in his bedroom, it turns out our concern was unnecessary. Jake is the most sober of them all. The family diplomat, often the only male in a household of women, he is prone to calling hotels home, as in "Let's go home, Dad," meaning to our hotel room. Long ago he picked up my habit of rearranging the hotel room furniture. He made his own way, and though he didn't take up a career in foreign affairs, he did follow me in this sense: he is making a living doing what he most loves.

Lorine is a young woman with a razor-sharp intellect and a tough, uncompromising, outspoken ethical sensibility. She did her postgraduate work in the field of sustainable development and practiced what she preached, often somewhat annoyingly. When her sister, Johanna, graduated with a photography degree from the University of the Arts in London, during the graduation ceremony there was a champagne toast for the graduates, and Lorine went around confiscating everyone's plastic flutes. "Come on, Lorine, it's your sister's graduation—that's going too far," I said. With a knowing smirk, Lorine promptly reached into her bag and pulled out half a dozen glass flutes to replace the plastic ones.

As our children were growing up, we traveled for pleasure frequently, though I seemed to have an infuriating (to Sheila) facility for finding stories wherever we went. During one safari to Zambia, we were camped out in tents in an area where a pride of lions prowled, and the guides kept warning us to be careful about leaving the tents to go to the latrine. That night Johanna was stricken with food poisoning, which we later discovered was because I had made her tuna fish sandwiches using mayonnaise that was three years out of date. I was up all night with her, helping her to the latrine about a hundred meters from her tent, both of us feeling exposed and vulnerable to the prowling lions, whose low growling seemed to surround us. It was both terrifying and deeply bonding.

The only good thing about food poisoning is that it is swift in its retribution; twenty-four hours with a young and healthy person, and it is usually finished. So we were able to continue our safari along the Zambezi River, just upstream from the Victoria Falls, the largest waterfall in Africa and one of the most stupendous in the world. We had moved from the bush to a posh hotel in Livingstone that catered to high-end tourists.

Sheila went off on a photo safari by herself while I watched the kids, after promising not to work. Lorine came running into our camp, beside herself with excitement, to tell me that she had seen a group of tourists gathered by the riverside because elephants were being swept downstream and falling over the Victoria Falls to their deaths. "Dad, you've got to do a story on this," she said. "This is huge!"

And she was right, it was a great story. Lorine then got her siblings involved, and the kids all badgered me to work on it—overruling my protests that we were on vacation, so I shouldn't work, as their mother had insisted. They were still quite young, so I just took them with me on the reporting. They got to see what journalism was like up close and experience it themselves. Together the four of us went to the game warden's office to interview him about this phenomenon of elephants getting washed over the falls. I thought, only in Africa could I do something like this—one of the reasons I've always loved working on the continent. During the interview, Jake, who couldn't have been older than five, sat in my lap. Meanwhile, as I conducted the interview, Lorine, then ten, sat next to me, poking me and whispering that I should ask tougher questions.

That was never my modus operandi. I always thought you got a lot more by gaining the subject's confidence and drawing the story out of them, rather than trying to confront them about it. The game warden explained that Zimbabwe shared the Zambezi River border with Zambia, so just across the river in Zimbabwe, the government had again begun to allow hunters to come and hunt elephants, something that had been banned in most countries and in Zimbabwe for many years. Because of this, the elephants were fleeing Zimbabwe by crossing the Zambezi River along a path that they remembered from decades earlier, going from large stone to large stone and swimming in between, in the almost hopeless way that elephants swim. It seems like they are far more likely to sink in the process, but they do manage to make headway. Slowly.

Now, they knew these pathways from many years past, thanks to that elephantine memory of theirs. But they didn't know that on the Zambian side, there was now a luxury hotel—the one that we were staying in—whose managers wanted to make sure crocodiles didn't climb up the banks, startle the tourists, or even attempt to lunch with their guests. So the hotel had installed electrified fencing along the banks of the river. The elephants ran into it, received a shock, and therefore turned back, exhausted from climbing the banks and swimming across the river once. Many just could not cope and gave up. Thus, they were washed over the falls—as many as one hundred of them, the warden confirmed, thanks to my demanding daughter who kept asking the game warden point-blank, "How many?"

It was indeed a memorable story, and Lorine took a picture of the scene on the riverbank as people were watching the elephants get washed over. (The photograph was later published in *Newsweek*'s online edition.) For once, my kids had an opportunity to see what exactly it was that their father did in all these countries he visited. My son observed, "This doesn't look very difficult really."

And in a way he was right.

Except when it came to covering war.

"DEATH OF A VILLAGE"
Newsweek
April 14, 1996

The villagers gathered in small groups to watch a video we had made of their destroyed hometown. They all wanted to see the evidence with their own eyes, and despite the anticipated devastation, they wanted another, nostalgic glimpse of Lehovici. The children were delighted to recognize the spring, the streams, the pastures they had played in. Their parents burst into tears at the sight of their ruined homes, even though they expected as much, but they gasped with relief at the one piece of news the video brought them: "Look," said one villager, "the cemetery hasn't been destroyed." Headstones dating from Ottoman times were still intact, and the refugees could discern the more recent graves of loved ones.

The kids especially were delighted to recognize the tan mongrel we saw on our first visit. One shouted: "That's Redzep's dog!" Redzep Hasanovic, one of the missing villagers, was the tallest man in Lehovici by a whole head; beside his now burned-down house was a basketball hoop on a grass court. His teenage children are all taller than 6 feet already, even 16-year-old daughter Ermina. "Let us go back there," said his wife, Sadeta. "To look for them, or at least for their bodies." Zina Hasanovic, whose husband's body shielded Mevludin, had no hope of finding her spouse alive, but still she wanted to go back to the Srebrenica enclave. "Now I want to be able at least to see the mass grave," she said. "To know where he is. And to show Lejla so that she'll know where her father is." Even that minimal act of closure is still denied to the villagers. They may not get any peace of mind until the ground finishes giving up its dead and the world finds a way to punish the murderers.

CHAPTER 10

The Sarajevo of the Mind

It was a European war.

Indeed, for much of it, I basically commuted to the war from my home in Rome at the other side of the Italian peninsula. I would drive across the Apennines, north to Ancona, a port city on the Adriatic. There I was able to catch the regular NATO supply flight heading into Sarajevo, in the international community's effort to relieve the Serb siege of the Bosnian capital. I did the same in reverse, so on many weekends I was able to get home to Sheila and our growing family.

The brutal Siege of Sarajevo from 1992 to 1996 went on for most of those four years—longer than the siege of Stalingrad—and presented daunting challenges for those of us who covered it. We would return to our rooms at the Holiday Inn in Sarajevo, a fifteen-story modern aluminum-and-glass edifice on the aptly named Sniper Alley, the main boulevard through Sarajevo. Serb snipers were perched in houses and on the mountainside opposite, and they fired at pretty much everything that moved. The hotel building itself was also frequently shelled. When it was particularly bad, I'd drag all the bedding into the bathtub and hunker down at the most interior point of the room possible.

The group of French photographers staying in the hotel were contemptuous of my war reporter philosophy: only stupid people aren't afraid. I didn't win them over with my jokes, one of which went like this:

Question: What's the best mine detector when you head down the road?

Answer: A French photographer.

We journalists would always wear body armor in the much-shelled Holiday Inn. Back then this armor was quite heavy. The vest that I wore weighed something like thirty pounds, with ballistic plates inserted in pouches front and back. Our rooms were on the seventh floor, so the climb up with all that gear was challenging, an unmatched Stairmaster. It was also a good way of keeping fit; not since my boxing days had I been in such good shape.

We spent a tremendous amount of energy simply figuring out how to get from one place to another safely. Our insurance policy, so to speak, was an armored Land Rover that *Newsweek* and its parent company, the *Washington Post*, shared. An experience comparable to sharing a romantic partner—never a good idea and almost always doomed to failure. Like many of the armored cars in those days, ours was up-armored, meaning it had armor plates added to a normal vehicle, the Land Rover. The plates were far too heavy for the suspension and the drivetrain of the vehicle. This system did stop most small arms fire, although we were keenly aware that it could not even come close to protecting us from the Serbs' .50 caliber Russian sniper rounds. The simplest of actions—such as going back to the hotel after a hard day's work—felt like something out of an action film. We would tear down Sniper Alley at breakneck speed, make a sudden left just past the Holiday Inn, out of the snipers' sights at least briefly, to the street behind it, which we would then go down and jump the curb into a grassy area behind the hotel, at which point we would be out of sight of the snipers again. Then we would swerve to the left again, jumping another curb onto a ramp down to the safety of the underground garage. The heavy metallic sound of sniper rounds striking our armored car has stuck with me my whole life—any one of those rounds could have succeeded in piercing the armor or finding a weak point, which gratefully never happened. But it's fair to say that I've never been shot at quite so much and quite so personally as in Sarajevo.

The Serbs did, of course, hit many people, ranging from children to elderly pedestrians, because they were indiscriminate in their targets. At the same time, the Siege of Sarajevo was front and center in the world's news agenda, and the Sarajevans inspired much admiration for the way they met the crisis with great good spirit, often with art and theater—always with defiance.

It was dangerous throughout the entire Balkan region. One evening in Croatia, just over the northern Bosnian border, I was in my hotel room getting ready to go to bed when someone from the management knocked on the door. "Get out of the room, get into the hallway now," he said urgently. "They're walking their mortars down the row of buildings, and it looks like this building will be next." I did as he suggested and was in the hallway just when a mortar round hit the room I had been in. Everything was destroyed, including the bed in which I would have been resting; there was a big gaping hole in the wall and the window was entirely missing. Potentially lethal shards of glass were scattered everywhere. (Nothing in a blast is more deadly than flying glass.)

Three years after the Srebrenica Massacre, when seven to eight thousand men and boys were massacred in cold blood and dumped into mass graves or buried using earth-moving equipment, the photographer Gary Knight and I went into the Srebrenica enclave and focused on Lehovici, a single village. If we focused on one community, we thought, we could make what had happened seem much more real and understandable to readers. We went door to door in Lehovici, visited every house—there were about twenty-five of them—much like census takers, trying to determine if any men were left alive and to find out, to the extent possible, what had happened to them. In addition to sneaking across Serbian lines around the Srebrenica enclave to reach the village, we used a handheld video camera—this was long before the days of smartphones. Then we somehow managed to gather a crowd of women from Lehovici from their refuge in camps around Tuzla in northern Bosnia, then under government control, and with a portable little TV monitor, we set up in a large hall and played for each family the videos of their homes; it was gut-wrenching for them and for us.

By 1995, the evidence of Serbian atrocities had mounted to such a degree that NATO, after years of threatening air strikes against the Serbs, finally began carrying them out, in a week-long campaign that bombed targets from Belgrade to Pale in Bosnian Serb territory. The NATO air strikes provided us with the perfect opportunity to cross the mountains between Albania and Kosovo, which was then Serb-held territory and is now semi-independent. Once into Kosovo, we had complete freedom of movement and were able to start looking at some of the atrocities that had occurred there because of the level of hatred between Albanians and Serbs. Most of the victims were ethnically Albanian. There were quite a few instances of atrocities, but what stood out in my mind more than anything was the multigenerational massacre in the village of Suva Reka, where an entire extended family of fifty people, young children and all, had been killed only because they were Albanians.

The long war in Yugoslavia, a hideously pointless and violent episode, became the place that many long friendships were made. For me, one in particular was with Alissa Rubin, who was then based in Vienna with the *L.A. Times*. Bosnia was her first war zone—she would soon cover many and win a Pulitzer for her work in Afghanistan. But this was where she cut her teeth as a war correspondent, and I could see that she had the instincts to become a great one. By two wars and many travails later, she had become my BFF.

Alissa and I first met when fighting over a fixer, Zoran Cirjakovic, who was easily the best in Yugoslavia. He was a Serb who was very critical of other Serbs. Thanks to *Newsweek*'s far more generous foreign news budget, I had more money, but she had known him much longer and had won his loyalty. Alissa and I ended up working something out so we could both use him. Happily, our tussle over Zoran's invaluable services turned into a deep friendship that endured through many war zones. Over the course of our careers, she was my boss twice, and I was hers once. And we each, in different ways, saved each other's life (Alissa was there when I woke up in the hospital after my medevac flight from India).

Like all the truly great fixers, Zoran understood how to get things done under nearly every possible circumstance. If we needed a translator, a local contact, a driver, an official in the government or the military, a car, or a place to stay, we only had to ask Zoran, and in his quiet and supremely competent fashion, he would make it happen.

Fixers are some of the most essential people on the planet for foreign correspondents. In war zones, it is not foreign correspondents who get killed, not usually; it is far more likely to be the fixers, assistants, translators, and other locals working for them. The Committee to Protect Journalists has been recording the deaths of journalists and media workers since 1992 worldwide, and most of them were either local reporters or locals working as fixers for foreign media. When foreign journalists are kidnapped, often their local drivers and translators are killed out of hand, while they are held to be ransomed off. When the foreign correspondents have finished working in a particular area, the locals usually have to remain behind—and often pay the price from hostile governments or individuals who can do little to the foreign correspondents, but anything they want to the locals.

For many years, foreign journalists carried body armor and helmets into war zones but expected the locals who accompanied them not to wear any protection. Journalists arrived with extensive training in hostile environments, courses that have become prerequisites for working in war zones, but there was none of that for the local staff, who often were hired merely because they spoke English, not because of any experience on the front lines. Among the foreign press, as with the military and their terps (interpreters), there has long been a double standard about the value of human life. The story I am proudest of from my years in Sarajevo did not win any big awards. Back in New York from a turn in Sarajevo, *Newsweek* editor Mark Whitaker told me to write a piece that would sum up my experience in Sarajevo. "Write it how you want to, with feeling. Write as if you're seeing it from 20,000 feet." This last sentence was a favorite expression of editors, especially at *Newsweek*, which had made such stories its trademark. The result was the following piece, which I look back on as one of the best I ever published:

"COUNTING THE DEAD, IN THE
SARAJEVO OF THE MIND"
By Rod Nordland
Newsweek, January 24, 1994

Every age has a city whose predicament defines its times, like Berlin in the 1950s or Saigon in the 70s or Beirut in the 80s. Sarajevo, whose airlift has outlasted Berlin's and whose casualties outnumber Beirut's, is the symbol for the 90s. The cold war is over, the world united against an ethnic aggressor whose acts have made it universally loathsome, but still the international community proves unable to act. Once again last week NATO repeated its threats of air strikes against the Serbs if they don't let up.

The Serbs continued a bombardment heavier than any in the war so far. "Sarajevans will not be counting the dead," Bosnian Serb leader Radovan Karadzic cawed in a speech to his rump parliament last week. "They will be counting the living." President Clinton tried to sound tough, while acknowledging how many times the allies had already backed off. "We should not say things that we do not intend to do." No one under the guns was convinced. "Air strikes are fairy tales we tell our children," says a Bosnian soldier.

Sarajevo isn't a rough place like some of its metaphoric predecessors; it has a European familiarity they lacked. Urbane and well-educated, Sarajevans keep producing culture in nights illuminated by the candles we distribute, heated by the crude wood stoves we pass out. Our capitals parade the fruits of an enduring intellectual life: a film series in New York, a new play in London, a children's art exhibit at the Georges Pompidou Center in Paris. We heap kudos on its still-publishing newspaper, *Oslobodjenje*, and hail its 13-year-old diarist Zlata Filipovic as a modern-day Anne Frank.

For a while, such attention inspired hope; now a war-weary cynicism replaces it. "Somewhere there is always a show for the world to watch," says Dr. Bakir Nakas, director of the city's State Hospital. Last Thursday two rockets blasted his hospital's 10-story facade; the evidence could scarcely be discerned among 500 other shell holes. "Some years it is Palestine, some years it is Iraq. This year it is here," Nakas says. VIP visits and solidarity meetings begin to wear thin; the motivation behind them, transparent. "They do it only to clear their consciences," says theater producer Aida Cengic.

All the admiration in the world can't change the quotidian reality on Sarajevo's streets. The sun comes out, the kids go out to play, the Serb gunners target playgrounds. Their intentions

are clear, their marksmanship honed by 21 months of practice—
more than half the children shot by snipers are wounded in the
head. "If the war continues for another 20 months, at the present rate, everyone in Sarajevo will have been wounded at least
once," says pediatric surgeon Salahudin Dizdarevic. That's an
exaggeration, but not by much; some 60,000 have now been
wounded out of 300,000 remaining residents. Aida Smailhodzic,
a 30-year-old gymnastics coach for the Bosnian national team,
was blown off her feet by a shell that hit in front of her building
last Tuesday. "I can't bear it anymore," she said from her hospital ward. "It's driving me crazy. It would be easier if they said,
'We will kill them all at once,' rather than like this, slowly."

The U.N. Protection Force has done little to help. Recently
a *Newsweek* reporter happened across a group of six badly
wounded civilians. They had dragged one another into an alleyway for shelter after a shell exploded among them as they
walked home from their jobs at midafternoon. The reporter, Joel
Brand, watched as two French armored personnel carriers came
by, paused to look, and sped away. One of the wounded men had
already lost a leg from an earlier shelling. Elsewhere, U.N. armored vehicles escort trash crews and distribute big white U.N.
bins for the shell debris; lately, heavily guarded U.N. engineers
have been repairing the city's trolley line, which runs right up
the middle of the perilous Snipers Alley. Sarajevans, who rarely
hide their contempt for the United Nations, don't even bother
to laugh at such efforts any longer.

The international community can only grasp at improbable
solutions. The International Rescue Committee, an American
aid group, is building a water-treatment plant inside a secret
mountain tunnel to protect it from Serb shells. The International Committee of the Red Cross's soup kitchens for the elderly offer take-home service, so that concentrations of hungry

diners won't attract a mortar attack. A French group, Solidarités, is planning a mobile books-and-crafts project, to keep kids occupied and off the streets; it will feature the world's first armored bookmobile. "Maybe we should provide all the kids with helmets and flak jackets, as well," says Solidarités official Dianne Cullinane, only half joking.

Writer Zlatko Dizdarevic calls Sarajevo "a city that refuses to die." This is no longer an optimism widely shared. "Every day the pool gets smaller, every day the odds get worse," says theater producer Cengic. "It's like bingo," says Lejla Canic, a 22-year-old law student whose boyfriend was recently killed. "Everyone has a number—'B 37,' and you're dead." Ten dead, 42 wounded last Wednesday; 11 dead, 62 wounded Thursday; 3 dead, 16 wounded Friday; and so on. Unless something changes, Sarajevo will be remembered as the place where the world just watched as number after number came up on the board.

"DANGEROUS DAYS"
Newsweek
February 1, 2002

In scrawled handwriting on a page torn from a reporter's notebook, the
notice that went up at the conference room in Kabul's Intercontinental
Hotel late last November was a *cri de coeur*. "Bad News. Our beloved
colleague and friend is dead. Ulf Stromberg, news cameraman for TV4
Sweden was shot dead . . ."

Ulf had opened the door of his room in a house in Taloqan, northern Afghanistan, and men in uniform had assassinated him under
somewhat mysterious circumstances. By then, the war had already
moved on to Kabul and other parts; Taloqan was a forgotten front and
most of the press there were already on their way out. Perhaps it was
just a last opportunity to pull off a robbery, but when Ulf reflexively
slammed the door shut, the gunmen opened fire. "Ulf lived for just
another 20 minutes," his colleagues wrote in the notice to the press
corps. "Our thoughts go to his wife Angela and his three lovely kids.
He was a hell of a cameraman. One of the greatest ever. We loved him.
Our sorrow is indescribable."

That sort of bad news became almost depressingly routine late last
year. Colleagues were picked off on the road to Kabul and on the front
lines outside of Khoja Bahawaddin, near the northernmost Tajikistan
border. Nearly all of those covering Afghanistan had used one of those
two routes in, and so it could have happened to anyone. By the end of
November, when eight Western journalists had been killed, the press
body count was higher than the American military's own death toll.

CHAPTER 11

At Two Wars

On September 11, 2001, I was in the garage of my house in Cobham, Surrey. Sheila and I had picked this location because after years of wandering around, it seemed important for our family to settle down and have a reliable center of geographical gravity. Sheila had a close friend in that particular suburb. I was then the chief foreign correspondent for *Newsweek* and the London bureau chief. I had converted the garage into a home office, and so on 9/11, I was working at home, with the television news on in the background, as usual.

And then, early in the afternoon (according to Greenwich mean time, of course), I glanced up and saw the "breaking news" chyron: a plane, American Airlines flight 11, had hit one of the World Trade Center towers. There was bewilderment and confusion: *Was this a stupid accident?* No. At 9:03 a.m. eastern standard time, another group of hijackers crashed United flight 175 into the South Tower, and a little more than half an hour later, at 9:37 a.m., American Airlines flight 77 crashed into the Pentagon. This was a coordinated attack of breathtaking scope and sophistication. I immediately got on the phone to the New York office of *Newsweek*, partly to make sure everyone there was OK and also to find out what I needed to do. No one knew—we were all scrambling to make sense of it, and in New York, obviously, the attack was personal. Offices in Midtown were being evacuated, but our staff was deployed to cover the scene of the wreckage.

I told Sheila to keep the kids away from the television (they were home from school that day)—already there was footage of people leaping out of buildings. And as I watched, I could see how traumatic this all would turn out to be. I said to myself, "Well, that's the end of Afghanistan as we know it." One of the few predictions I have made—something journalists should always avoid—that really came true.

I first booked a flight to Montreal, so I could drive down to New York and cover that end of the story. But the office told me that they had enough people there. Instead, I should be on the first plane that I could to Pakistan and get myself to Afghanistan as soon as possible. This is the unnatural life of a foreign correspondent; the rest of the world is told to sit still, "stay with your family." We are booking flights to get us as close to the lip of the active volcano as soon as possible.

When I went on my first foreign assignment, Gene Roberts told me that I should always travel with a blanket, a flask of alcohol, and a good book. Over the years, I had become a bit more sophisticated in what I carried in my backpack: my laptop, a satellite phone, my portable satellite internet transmitter, notebooks, extra batteries for everything, water purification tablets, a vessel to carry water (I came to like lightweight, expandable silicone bladders), and a small first-aid kit with morphine, which I discovered one could buy over the counter at pharmacies in some countries, such as Pakistan. And there's more. I like Olfa knives, little pocket tools with extractable blades, which are small and thin enough to be missed on airport x-ray machines. I like a space blanket—one side is reflective aluminum and the other thin flannel. It weighs barely three ounces, takes up very little room, and can be a lifesaver when it's cold and you are stuck somewhere. I make sure to bring several small, quick-drying microfiber towels, should I take a swim, or a shower in one of the crappy hotels journalists often end up staying in. I also carry a lightweight nylon sleeping cocoon, something to sleep in when the bed is too infested or dirty. My traveling coffee kit includes a week's supply of whole beans, a Japanese hand grinder, a collapsible silicone cup, a portable electric kettle the size of a pancake when stowed (or, for trips to places without electricity, a butane mini stove), a Ziploc bag of powdered whole milk, a fold-flat camping filter, but also, and finally, a clutch of no. 2 paper filters.

Naturally, I travel with large amounts of cash, for, well, everything from food to accommodations to bribing border guards. No, wait, I have never bribed a border guard; that would be a violation of US law, the Foreign Corrupt Practices Act, to be specific. One habit has often gotten me out of trouble: deep in the recesses or the lining of my wallet, I keep a rolled-tight hundred-dollar bill, often so well hidden it takes me a while to find it. That's not much of a backup these days—a hundred bucks won't go very far anymore, but it'll get you to or from the airport in most towns. I also used to carry a Halo or Everlit sucking-chest-wound dressing—it's thin, takes up little space, and one never knows . . . Sucking chest wounds often occur when the body is pierced by a bullet or piece of shrapnel. Such a wound is identifiable by its audible sucking noise; it is life threatening if not immediately sealed. I fervently hoped never to use such a dressing, nor the Bic pen in my kit, kept there in case an injured person stopped breathing due to a blocked airway. You can use the pen to perform an emergency tracheotomy, in a crude but effective manner. Emergency interventions like this one are taught in hazardous-environment first-aid courses, to prepare you for what to do if a proper trauma center cannot be reached within the Golden Hour—the precious stretch of time during which most victims can be saved, if transported to a trauma center. Civilian first aid is aimed at stabilizing the victim for the trip to the nearest hospital. Hazardous-environment first aid takes over if no such facility is within reach.

I raced for the first flight to Islamabad, which would require a visa to Pakistan. Every foreign correspondent in Pakistan at the time was angling to get a visa to Afghanistan. The Taliban government kept leading us along, saying they would process our visa requests in another day or two.

Finally, a group of us organized our own transportation, visas be damned, in cars and a minibus, to travel down the perilous highway over the Khyber Pass to Kabul, known during British rule as the Grand Trunk Road. Today it's a modern though extremely treacherous two-lane road carved out of the mountainside, with lots of sharp turns alongside a deep gorge. The road is not only dangerous because of its many switchbacks. Ambushes are often staged from the mountain slopes above it. The boulder-strewn sides of the gorge are littered with burned and rusted cars, buses, trucks, and even old Soviet tanks that didn't make it.

Once out of the Khyber Pass, at the Afghan border, we passed the smoking wreckage of a car that had been caught in a Taliban ambush. Six Spanish journalists inside were killed. Our car had been only a mile behind theirs. I deserve no credit for surviving that trip—it was just dumb luck. Years later, when I ran bureaus in Kabul, I would never have deemed a trip like that one safe, and I often overruled use of that route for our reporters. When we saw the Spaniards' car that day, I had my driver turn and go back to Peshawar.

There I caught a ride with the Mine Action Group, an NGO with the goal of locating and removing land mines. This trip too seemed star-crossed. We stopped for lunch in Jalalabad, at a dubious-looking kebab joint. I ate something that gave me a case of food poisoning unlike any I had ever experienced. I spent a few days in my hotel room, crawling to the toilet and back to the bed while suffering the twin afflictions of diarrhea and vomiting. Finally, an Afghan doctor was summoned and announced he was going to give me an injection. The Afghan health-care system generally prefers injections to pharmaceuticals. No matter what ails you, an injection provides the cure. Though sick, I had the presence of mind to notice that the doctor had no alcohol swabs and that his hands were filthy, so I told my friends to keep him away.

On October 7, 2001, the US-led coalition of British and American forces began Operation Enduring Freedom.

I had covered Afghanistan since the *Inquirer* sent me there in 1979, on the heels of the Soviet invasion. This was during the Cold War, of course, so easing into the country as a Western reporter required a bit of subterfuge—in retrospect it seems the stuff of a Peter Sellers comedy. Several other journalists and I went to Kabul and posed as rug buyers. We stayed at the Intercontinental Hotel, an improbable five-star joint in a town full of one- and two-star dumps. When the authorities grew suspicious, they put us under house arrest. We were stuck in the hotel for the duration of the invasion. Though finally released and sent on our way, we didn't manage to do the reporting we had hoped for. But we came home with plenty of Afghan carpets, and we at least could claim the dateline.

I made up for that superficial initial exposure to Afghanistan over the following years—from 1994 to 2001 when the Taliban was in power, and then covering the war for nearly twenty years after the US invasion. On one of my earliest reporting trips, during the jihadi war against the Soviets, I traveled in the mountains with twenty mujahideen under Commander Abdul Haq. The trip was reminiscent of my trek with the Contras in Nicaragua in terms of physical demands: bad food and embedding with some often-unpleasant insurgents.

That trip also laid the foundation for my lifelong dislike for the dominant culture of Afghan men. I was with Abdul Haq's unit in the mountains of eastern Kunar Province, not far from the border with Pakistan, watching as they tried to lay the groundwork for incursion. But the most significant event for me was the capture of a teenage Russian soldier. He must have been around eighteen, maybe nineteen years old when taken prisoner. Commander Haq basically treated him as his sex slave, raping him every night in his tent, to loud guffaws from the other guys.

Under any circumstances, this behavior would be considered repulsive. But for me, the son of a convicted pedophile who raped children, to be present yet unable to intervene was nearly unbearable. As an *Inquirer* reporter assigned to accompany these men, I was in an impossible situation. I could not have done anything effective. Neither was I psychologically astute enough to be aware of how triggering—to use contemporary trauma vocabulary—this experience must have been for me. I recall lying in my sleeping bag, coiled with rage and helplessness. Still, I learned something. I saw the kind of men these mujahideen were, their character and their lack of morality, and I loathed them both individually and collectively.

One night I sat at the campfire, having a long talk with Commander Haq and trying to persuade him not to kill the young captive. Our conversation went downhill after he asked me about what, to him, was a shocking American practice: that a woman can divorce her husband. This was unheard of in Afghanistan's patriarchy, among all its many factions, until many years of American presence and the efforts of women's rights activists of the international community. Haq found the notion of female-initiated divorce infuriating. As I often do, in this moment I overshared, telling him my own mother had divorced my father because of physical abuse. Big mistake. That's when I first heard the repulsive motto of the Afghan patriarchy: "Beat your wife every day; if you don't know what she did, she will."

I spent many hours that night trying to win him over, but Commander Haq was no fool. "I know you're trying to talk me out of killing that infidel, but it'll never work." I had noticed the commander covetously eyeing my Swiss Army knife, and in a land where life is cheap, I thought I might offer the knife to him in exchange for the prisoner's life. He jumped at the offer and took my knife; we shook hands on the deal, and later he came back for the knife's leather belt pouch. Afghans were, usually, men of honor where their word was concerned. In this way they were often reliable. "I promise I won't kill the infidel," he'd said when he pocketed the knife, putting it in his baggy Pashtun-style trousers.

After another couple days' march, we stopped at the margins of what the muj figured was a Soviet minefield. Their prisoner was an officer of some sort—probably the Soviet equivalent of a freshly minted second lieutenant, since he was so young. The Afghans interrogated him roughly, slapping him around, but he insisted his unit had had nothing to do with laying mines there and that he had no idea where they were. They put him on point, guns trained at his back. He crept so slowly, knowing each step could be his last; watching his tentative progress and recalling the abuse he suffered made me unbearably sad. We lost sight of him as he passed over a slight rise, then soon we heard an explosion. The mujahideen thought this was hilarious. The commander said, "Well, I guess he was telling the truth." Which evoked another round of laughter. "Can you believe it?" It was hard not to detest these men. Later we followed the Russian POW's trail until we came across his mangled young body, the comical Soviet officer's high-crowned, broad-brimmed hat lying off to one side. Then we veered off into heavy woods, which were safer than the open terrain of the minefield. In later years the widespread glorification of the mujahideen in Afghanistan and much of the Western world made my skin crawl.

Later the muj sold me (for a hundred dollars) a broken-down packhorse to ride back to Pakistan. I rode up to Commander Haq's tent, dismounted, and demanded, "What about our deal?"

He replied amiably: "I promised that *I* couldn't kill him and *I* didn't; the Russians who set those mines did." There was no sense in arguing the point with him.

Newsweek's end-of-the-week deadline was fast approaching, and I badly wanted to file that story—so badly that I pushed that horse so hard, he dropped dead at the end of the trail (he already looked halfway dead when I first mounted him, poor creature). I was trying to feed and water him when this happened; he just sank to his front knees and gave up breathing. Somehow I got back to Peshawar just in time to file, but *Newsweek* couldn't use the story, due to some huge story that day somewhere else in the world that I do not remember.

The mujahideen consisted of a group of warlord-run brotherhoods who terrorized Afghanistan—and one another. Kabul was shelled by rival gangs, and this left the city, and the whole country really, craving anything that resembled order. The Taliban brought them this. They quickly rose to power in 1996, suppressing the warlords and thereby becoming wildly popular. They restored daily life to something resembling normalcy, though at a high price: they took away women's rights.

Before their rule, you could see women wearing miniskirts in the streets of Kandahar. When the Taliban took power, they would whip people in the street if their clothing was what they considered indecent. "Indecent" did not mean anything as provocative as cleavage; it meant showing an elbow. They closed schools for women and decreed that none would be allowed to work, except as doctors. Women were allowed to go only to female doctors—though barely a handful were available in the whole country. This was especially cruel; many war widows from the time of the Soviet conflict needed to earn a living to support their large families. They were fired from their jobs and in many cases reduced to near starvation.

What can you say about a country with a vice president who, as recently as 2021, was famous for using two dwarfs as hood ornaments, dressing them up in military gear to ride on the hood of his

Humvee everywhere he went. This is General Abdul Rashid Dostum, the same general accused of repeatedly raping and torturing the elderly male politicians who crossed him. As one of his former bodyguards told me, on the record, Dostum also murdered his first wife, the mother of two of his children, in a fit of rage over an imagined transgression. He denied this, saying she had grabbed an AK-47 stowed behind a fridge and set it off by mistake, shooting herself repeatedly in the chest and head—an act of bodily contortion almost impossible to imagine.

In the early 1950s, a young journalist and soon-to-be-novelist named James Michener spent a year in Afghanistan, producing a novel called *Caravans*. He crisscrossed the country, and already the great game was on between the United States and the Soviets. The Soviets were building "model farms" in Jalalabad; the Americans were draining the marshes of Helmand and introducing sophisticated large-scale irrigated cultivation, modeled on the Tennessee Valley plan. At a key point in Michener's book, an American and a Russian are confronted by a savvy Afghan, who says to them, "You Americans and you Russians, you're both going to invade my country and you're both going to be really sorry for it." Mind you, this was published in 1963.

The escalation of Operation Enduring Freedom consumed my attention during the early 2000s. I was practically a commuter between Kabul and our family home. I'd spend several weeks on the ground—Alissa Rubin once said that eight weeks was the maximum amount of time one could be deployed to these areas without suffering from overload. Throughout the escalation of the conflict, I watched the Americans bring in their raft of consultants and their troops, make attempts at creating an infrastructure. I had a ringside seat at the creation of a tragedy. But the stories were everywhere, and I attacked them with the urgency the situation seemed to demand: the generals and their ambitions, the troops on the ground and their realities, the people of Afghanistan adjusting to this new collection of authority figures imposed upon them. I saw girls begin to get educated again, while families and warlords hardened their commitment to old traditions. The bellicose triumphalism of President George W. Bush and his cronies was juxtaposed with the Taliban's determination not to surrender. It was a quagmire in the making. Michener's observation was playing out in real time.

Then, of course, Iraq happened. Bush, unable to contain himself, led a coalition looking for bogus weapons of mass destruction and invaded Iraq, first by air on March 19, 2003, and then with ground troops the next day. Bush triumphantly declared the "end of major combat operations" on May 1, 2003, though US troops remained in Iraq until 2011.

I worked in Iraq before Saddam Hussein fell, while he was falling, and after he fell. A decade and more after the American invasion, I was still making trips there, and not because I liked it. In fact, I never liked it—what was there to like? It ruined my marriage, my family relations, and from time to time, my health. But for a journalist, Iraq was simply too compelling and too important a place to avoid, especially from 2003 to 2009, when I pretty much lived there full time.

My first visits to Iraq took place in the early 1980s, before anything like Google existed. Journalists could curate a selection of our clips in such a way that we appeared to offer a sympathetic ear, and thus gain access to the country. Once search engines came along, those in power in Iraq knew within seconds exactly who you were, and what you thought. My earliest trip to the country took place during the Iran-Iraq War, which lasted from 1980 until 1988. Our government minders were with us constantly and took us to the battlefield in southern Iraq near Basra, where, they claimed, the Iranians had just launched a poison gas attack against Iraqi forces—an accusation that each side often made about the other. Indeed, both may have been culpable.

At that battlefield near Basra, dead bodies were scattered everywhere. Some of them were already swelling, and most were either wearing or carrying gas masks. It was a scene of such unimaginable loss and suffering, and yet, in the midst of it, our Iraqi minders set up a long table for our lunch—lamb chops, roasts, kebabs—in the middle of this horrific and fetid landscape.

At the start of the war, I set up the *Newsweek* bureau, and then, when I was hired by the *New York Times* in 2009, I joined their enormous operation. Running bureaus in that environment—where security was such an enormous challenge—was a complicated and many-layered undertaking. At *Newsweek* we shared premises with the *Los Angeles Times* and the *Wall Street Journal*. Alissa Rubin was still at the *L.A. Times*, and together we decided to find a place for our teams within the Green Zone—a perimeter of safety that some journalists criticized us for choosing, suggesting that it placed us too close to the locus of power. We found this argument ludicrous: of course, we were going to cover all these stories as rigorously as possible, and many of them would be about power. Hubris and grandiloquence thrived in Iraq like nowhere else.

Key to keeping safe in both Iraq and Afghanistan was a fleet of expensive security advisers—mostly men in their forties and fifties who had previous military experience in elite special forces or marine units. Some were from the British Royal Marines or had retired from American Special Forces; all were looking for that last big score. In those days these advisers, especially those who worked in "close protection" roles—which meant actual bodyguards for dignitaries or officials—could earn as much as a thousand dollars a day. We also had Iraqi bodyguards: some accompanied us on reporting "missions" while others served as stationary guards on the walls and roofs of our compounds. Such 24/7 coverage added up to a lot of personnel, and someone had to manage them, which meant managing men with guns.

One night the *Wall Street Journal* and *Newsweek* staff, occupants of the same building, threw a party for journalists, westerners from NGOs, and others who were working in Baghdad. Flying in the face of well-established rules, the *Newsweek* security adviser, Derek, was drinking and began to play a game of darts with *Wall Street Journal* correspondent Philip Shishkin, who was a great player. He cleaned Derek's clock, which so infuriated Derek that, after losing a match, he put the barrel of his 9mm automatic revolver against Philip's head and threatened to blow his brains out. "Say your prayers and prepare to die, motherfucker," Derek shouted, which did not sound like a joke. Faced with such a threat, the intended victim commonly reacts by pissing their pants. But somehow Philip stayed incredibly calm, cool, collected . . . and dry. Derek's more sober, sensible friends pleaded with him to calm down and pulled him away from Philip, and the event passed without casualties—except Derek's career.

Derek's father, who had recommended his son to me for the job, was a legendary and much-feared RX Delta Force commando. When I summoned Derek the next morning, he came to the bureau with his hungover son. It was clear to everyone what I had to do, which was, of course, fire Derek. I was astonished that the father seemed surprised by that. He and Derek argued against it, on the grounds that the previous night's incident was really just a joke! And Derek was drunk. How could anyone consider this "good fun" a serious threat? Well, the *Wall Street Journal* reporter certainly could, as did I. "It's just unacceptable," I said to Derek, "and this is your last day on the job." Much protesting ensued, but I was not going to budge. Volatile alcoholic bullies could not be tolerated, especially to provide us with security.

It certainly turned out to be the right decision. A few months later the Iraqi authorities arrested Derek on charges of gun running.

They found an entire shipping container in the Green Zone packed full of weaponry, which Derek lamely claimed was for the use of *Newsweek*'s security staff—all six of us, I guess. The container held hundreds of M5 and AK-47 long rifles and Glock machine pistols, along with enough ammo for a small army. Obviously, he was trafficking them. Derek was a familiar type in war zones: a badge-heavy security adviser who would get into fights at the office. Drinking and guns are very dangerous companions, and there were several incidents in which security advisers killed several of their peers, or even some of their employers and their colleagues.

Running two wars at once was unsustainable, both for those of us covering them and for the overstretched American military. For a long time, things did not deteriorate in Afghanistan, and the country was relatively stable. But when the United States invaded Iraq, it poured all its resources there, at the cost of the forces in Afghanistan. By then suicide bombing as the weapon of choice changed everything. The combination of a distracted occupying force and the escalation of suicide bombing gave the Taliban a leg up. There have been suicide bombings in other countries and places—in Palestine and Israel they are seemingly part of daily life. But there had never been a systematic campaign of suicide bombings like the one in Afghanistan from 2005 on. And it made quite a difference in the war and the stability of the government.

I mentioned that each of my children is associated with a different war: Lorine, the eldest, with the beginning of the Bosnian conflict, Jo with the end of that conflict and the takeover of Afghanistan, and Jake with both Afghanistan and Iraq.

During that period, Sheila often complained that I was away too much, and that even when I was home, I wasn't really there—often I was working around the clock to run *Newsweek* bureaus in two war zones, Afghanistan and Iraq. They were big, demanding bureaus at work in dangerous, difficult times. Mentally, I was always there, and I had to be there—the lives of my staff members and fellow correspondents depended on the decisions I made and the guidance I gave.

I thought that I was managing to perform this juggling act as well as anyone could expect. When I had been in Sarajevo, running the *Newsweek* bureau when that story was front and center on the world stage, it was feasible, though not easy, to commute between Rome and Sarajevo every weekend. Then Iraq happened, and everything was so much harder. There was an eight-to-nine-hour time difference, and a commute home took twenty hours, requiring two to three long-haul flights. Like the American military in Iraq and Afghanistan, I was just absurdly overstretched, as much as I tried not to admit it—the generals rarely did either. But my juggling act—war correspondent, dad, and husband—was no longer sustainable. I often criticized the war effort with the line "Hope is not a plan." But if I'm to be honest, I have to admit that for all of us, whether in the military or in journalism, hope was all we had. In fact, we were betting on the come, and as in poker, that is usually a loser's hand.

Sheila and I, and all of America, were deep into two wars seemingly without end. *Newsweek* told me I was getting the promotion for which I had long lobbied, to the post of chief foreign correspondent.

By late 2008 *Newsweek* was imploding, and the rescue plan, in the face of financial disaster, was to cut the huge expense of foreign reporting, replacing journalism with inexpensive essays by academics and others for token "guest writer" fees. As the magazine's new chief foreign correspondent, I was told there would no longer be a travel budget, and I was henceforth to sit in London and produce essays reported, if at all, by phone. I immediately applied for a job at the *New York Times*, the only American news organization still investing heavily in foreign reporting. Meanwhile, the once great newsmagazine I had worked for throughout twenty years, in dozens of countries, was sold to a stereo magnate for one dollar and the assumption of its debt.

The *Times* had one possible opening, in Baghdad, where I knew many of the staff from my *Newsweek* days.

That was during the height of the Iraq War, in 2009, and the *New York Times* had the biggest bureau in Baghdad, which was also quite likely the biggest news bureau in the world at the time, possibly the biggest since Saigon in 1975. With an Iraqi staff of about 140 cooks, cleaners, drivers, translators, fixers, stringers, and security personnel, the bureau sometimes also employed as many as two dozen expats who worked as photographers, reporters, videographers, and producers. The guard force was large; we had to send bodyguards out with journalists whenever they went out on "missions"—as the security guys insisted on labeling our reporting trips. The *Times* bureau was an astonishing place, under the direction of John Burns and his wife, the late Jane Scott-Long. They carried out a million-dollar renovation of two adjoining villas, one to be used as a newsroom, and the other as accommodations for journalists—large bedrooms, all of them with en suite baths. This was nestled next to a newly dug swimming pool heated for winter and set in a pretty good approximation of an English garden, with clematis vines covering the inner walls and deep grassy lawns between them.

Yet the *New York Times* Baghdad bureau was infamous for its toxic atmosphere and sometimes violent intrigues, and I had long felt lucky to work in the far more congenial and friendly environment of *Newsweek*.

One day in 2008 one of the guards in the bureau came to Jane to tell her that the Iraqi security manager was conspiring with the guard staff to set up an ambush on the Airport Road the next day, when she was scheduled to fly home. She immediately called in the

British security manager and the Iraqi security manager and confronted them with the allegations.

The Iraqi security manager tried to laugh it off, saying they had only planned to fire guns in the air around Ms. Scott-Long's car as an innocent expression of protest over recent decreases in pay—supposedly to demonstrate how invaluable the guards were. Burns immediately fired the Iraqi security manager. But instead of supporting the decision, the British security manager tried to roll it back, on the grounds that there had been no serious threat. The Airport Road, called "Route Irish" by the military, was then the most dangerous stretch of road in Iraq, and probably the world. When the British security manager stuck up for his Iraqi subordinate, Burns fired him as well.

The problems in that bureau went beyond threats. One day Khalid, one of the Iraqi translators, was ambushed on his way to work. The attackers apparently had inside information, knew his route and timing, and were ready for him, opening fire on his car while he was waiting at a stoplight. He was unhurt in the first salvo but then made the tragic mistake of calling his mother on his cell phone. The attackers saw him move and came straight back to finish the job, killing Khalid while he was still on the phone with his mother.

I was aware of all this when I applied to the *Times* and discovered their only opening was in Baghdad, where they needed a temporary contractor, not a staffer. I decided to take the job, hoping to write my way into a staff position, which happened when they transferred me to Kabul as their deputy bureau chief there in 2011.

Simply getting from one place to another in Iraq and Afghanistan presented a complicated collection of problems. One option was a car—maybe even an armored one for extra safety. On the low-life pecking order, there are car salespeople, and then there are *armored car* salespeople. They are fond of throwing about terms like "bulletproof" or "blast proof" when in fact no such thing exists.

The only truly safe way to travel by armored car is for the subject (the principal, or the target, in the lingo of the security industry) to fill the armored car with bodyguards or other plausible decoys and then secretly travel by helicopter or just an anodyne civilian car instead. Even the armored car used by the president of the United States is reputedly armored only to Level B6+, meaning that it will stop most high-velocity rounds, including .50 caliber heavy machine-gun rounds—sort of. Furthermore, the armored glass will not have the same level of ballistic protection as the steel body, and the glass is unlikely to stop a .50 caliber bullet.

Typically, the ballistic armoring just applies to the passenger cabin of the vehicle, essentially creating a box of steel, Kevlar, and glass that offers enough resistance to protect the persons inside from a few bullets during an attack of relatively short duration. The armoring does not apply, or at least does not apply at quite such high a level, to the trunk and engine compartments, and certainly not to important accessories such as the wheels. It also does not offer any level of meaningful fire suppression, should accessories outside the armored box, such as the fuel tank, ignite. Plus, the rating as to the caliber of bullets fired applies only to one round hitting a given place in the armor, not, say, twenty or thirty rounds in a tight pattern hitting the same place.

Then there is the used armored car problem. Most civilian-use armored cars are in effect used cars; they are armored after manufacture, a process referred to as "up-armoring." As such, when the armor is added, key elements of their drivetrains and mechanical components will be subjected to stress and weight for which they were neither designed nor engineered. The armored car can easily weigh three or four times more than the original. Even if the brakes and suspension systems have been reinforced, as is usually the case, an up-armored car will not age well. It may look brand-new, since its mileage is low, but mechanical problems tend to be chronic. And on top of all that, the ballistic integrity of flexible armoring materials like Kevlar degrades with age—and does so especially quickly in a hot climate.

At one point during Mr. Burns's tenure, the *Times* Mercedes armored car needed serious engine repairs, and there were no qualified mechanics in Baghdad. The bureau actually FedExed the two-ton car to the nearest Mercedes dealer, in Kuwait City, and had it FedExed back, at something like $20,000 round trip.

If these cars are generally difficult to deal with, what about a helicopter? Proponents of helicopters like to point out that the civilian fatality rate from helicopter crashes is only slightly worse than that of fixed-wing aircraft. But that covers miles traveled in a car; helicopters are more likely to crash than cars based on hours traveled, or eighty-six times more likely based on miles traveled. Moreover, you are much more likely to survive a crash in a car than in a helicopter.

In an active war zone, the statistics are even worse, since generally speaking, in civilian life no one is trying to shoot down helicopters. But in Iraq, insurgents quickly got adept at doing this. The American military initially believed that the armoring on military helicopters would stop most small arms fire from penetrating the underside of the aircraft. Insurgents soon learned to set up overlapping fields of fire with several machine guns to find weak points above the armored undercarriage. Helicopters proved to be very dangerous in Iraq, accounting for nearly 10 percent of all American military fatalities during the first six years of the war. At the peak of the fighting, in 2007, seventeen helicopters were being hit a month. It became the practice for helicopters to fly in groups of at least two—chalk one and chalk two, as they would refer to themselves by radio—so that one helicopter could rescue the passengers of the other if it was hit.

Despite all that, helicopter use skyrocketed during the Iraq War, as the military greatly increased spending to purchase them and to train pilots. Helicopter air hours in Iraq went from 200,000 in 2004 to 400,000 by 2007. However dangerous helicopters were, by that time any sort of road travel in Iraq was far more so. Roadside bombs and IEDs (improvised explosive devices) were planted practically every block or two, hidden in piles of trash, in the bodies of road-killed dogs, in gutters and sewers, in a baby stroller left by the sidewalk. The same thing later happened in Afghanistan, where all trips for American diplomats from the US embassy to the international airport two miles away were made by helicopter. At one point American officials were using the huge Chinook helicopter literally to cross the street, from the embassy to Special Forces headquarters not two hundred yards away, at a fuel cost of $1,000 a passenger.

The danger of helicopters switched from theoretical to personal when my close friend Alissa Rubin was in an Iraqi Air Force helicopter when it crashed. She had hitched a ride to Mount Sinjar in Kurdistan, close to the Iraqi-Turkish border. The mountain is sacred to the Yazidi people, who had been targeted by ISIS as pagans and nonbelievers. ISIS was rounding up the women, enslaving them, and forcing them to provide sexual services or even to marry their recruits, actually auctioning them off in a marketplace. Alissa managed to get to the top of Mount Sinjar in that helicopter. The pilot was a general in the Iraqi Air Force with a big heart. Seeing the Yazidi refugees and knowing how dire their plight was, he let too many of them pile aboard, far above the helicopter's capacity. The pilot had trouble achieving lift with all that excess weight, so he decided to tilt the helicopter forward and fly off the edge of the mountain, using the drop-off to create lift. Then, he reasoned, once he was up in the air, he could carry on. But just as he started this maneuver, one of his skids caught on a rock, and the helicopter rolled and began tumbling down the mountainside. All the passengers ended up on top of Alissa, who suffered multiple major injuries as a result. Both her hands and wrists were crushed. One of her lungs

collapsed due to a chest injury. She had seven or eight fractures in
the skull, some of which would later require brain surgery.

On August 12, 2014, I filed a story with another *Times* reporter,
Rick Gladstone, the kind that one never wants to write. The headline
was "Crash of Rescue Helicopter Kills Pilot; Times Reporter Is
Injured."

When I initially had heard, on a Kurdish radio news bulletin,
that a helicopter had gone down with a female *New York Times*
reporter aboard, I knew it could only be Alissa Rubin. We had covered so many wars together over the previous twenty years, from
Bosnia and Kosovo to Afghanistan to Iraq and back again. She was
the colleague and friend I trusted the most, and I tend to think that
the feeling was mutual; we consulted each other constantly on the
many thorny security issues we faced. Of course we had disagree-
ments, but throughout, we always knew where the other one was,
and our friendship became a kind of protective shield no matter
where we went.

I did not hesitate to head to the Iraqi-Turkish border town of
Zakho, where we assumed correctly that ambulances would take any
survivors from the crash, since it was the nearest town with a proper
hospital. Kamel, who was one of our translators in Kurdistan—a
schoolteacher before he became a fixer, a wonderful man, very caring and decent—suggested that we drive all night to get there by
morning. It was a long drive through dodgy territory where ISIS was
known to be operating, but we got to the hospital in time to discover
that Alissa was in truly terrible shape but was being cared for in a
hospital at least.

There was a brain surgeon there, Kurdish but from Syria, and
he said that Alissa's injuries were so severe, she needed major brain
surgery. He said he could do this surgery himself, he felt he was
qualified, but the hospital did not have the facilities he would need

to do it properly. He recommended that we put all our energies into getting her medevacked to a decent hospital as soon as possible while he did what he could to stabilize her. I was fortunate because just as we arrived at the hospital, Sarah, a field producer from ITN TV, a British news outlet, was already there, trying to get a sense of what was going on. She briefed me quickly on where matters stood. Field producers are a unique breed in television. They are the ones who get nearly everything done: they prepare the reporters to go on camera, they get the names and the numbers and the details. They're journalists but they're also facilitators and fixers, and she had figured everything out, finding the phone numbers for the doctors in New York, for the insurance company that was going to pay for Alissa's medevac. Sarah was savvy and proactive in assuring that all was in order. The insurance company claimed that they had arranged for an ambulance to pick up Alissa, cross the Iraqi border into Turkey, and go to a private airport, where the medevac jet would meet Alissa. Sarah demanded the phone number of the ambulance driver. When the company couldn't provide it, this made Sarah suspect that no such arrangement had been made. She turned out to be correct.

In the end, with the help of the doctor, we took care of it ourselves. I have learned, from my own experience, that brain surgeons have a reputation for being macho and self-important—the arrogant rock stars of modern medicine. But this one proved himself to be a deeply caring man. He climbed into the ambulance with her, sat beside her, held her hand and reassured her, and then talked us through the Iraqi military customs and immigration checkpoints on the border, and similarly through the Turkish side as well.

We finally arrived in Turkey at a military airfield, where the medevac jet met us, with a doctor and nurse aboard. The plane had a long, slim fuselage just wide enough for a stretcher and someone to sit or kneel next to it, and that is where I positioned myself. "Am

I going to die?" Alissa asked me. If I had told her the truth, I would have said, "You certainly look like you are going to die." But I assured her that no such thing was going to happen, even though I didn't believe it myself.

Turkey is a big country, and it was a long flight to Istanbul. We were bound for the American hospital there and its intensive care unit. There, the medical team worked to stabilize Alissa but not to operate on her brain. The plan was to get her to New York, to the Weill Cornell Medical Center. There, its storied brain surgeon, Dr. Phil Stieg, had agreed to take her case on an emergency basis.

There are few friendships quite so intense as those forged among colleagues in war zones. Many credited me with saving Alissa's life by getting her out of Zakho safely, but I deserve only a portion of the credit. Just as much belongs to the Kurdish brain surgeon; my heroic driver, Kamil, who drove me overnight through known ISIS territory; the British field producer, Sarah, who detected and unraveled the insurance company's fuckup of the medevac plans for Alissa; and of course Dr. Stieg. Then, just five years later, it was Alissa's turn to return the favor, and she did so in spades. One of the many things she made happen was to persuade Dr. Stieg to open up his busy surgical schedule, populated with billionaires and VIPs, slip me into it, and operate on me almost immediately after I arrived at Weill Cornell. Since then Alissa has been kind of a guardian angel, hovering over my treatment and care, making sure to keep me safe. I once heard someone say that if you save someone's life, you will be in it forever. Her sister Hannah once said to me, out of the blue, "You're a member of our family now. Without a Rod there wouldn't be an Alissa. And without an Alissa—and a Leila and a Stieg—there wouldn't be a Rod."

Somehow, this story—Alissa's brain injuries from a helicopter crash, and mine from a "space-occupying lesion," both of us just doing our jobs in places far from home when our lives instantly became unrecognizable, and both of us ending up on Dr. Stieg's operating table—illustrates a kind of symmetry to our work as foreign correspondents. Something connects us: these strange places, the intensity of every day, the front-row seats in the theater of history, and that smoldering sense of invulnerability, which can be extinguished in an instant.

"2 STAR-CROSSED AFGHANS CLING TO LOVE, EVEN AT RISK OF DEATH"
New York Times
March 9, 2014

BAMIAN, Afghanistan—She is his Juliet and he is her Romeo, and her family has threatened to kill them both.

Zakia is 18 and Mohammad Ali is 21, both the children of farmers in this remote mountain province. If they could manage to get together, they would make a striking couple.

She dresses colorfully, a pink head scarf with her orange sweater, and collapses into giggles talking about him. He is a bit of a dandy, with a mop of upswept black hair, a white silk scarf, and a hole in the side of his saddle-toned leather shoes. Both have eyes nearly the same shade, a startling amber.

They have never been alone in a room together, but they have publicly declared their love for each other and their intention to marry despite their different ethnicities and sects. That was enough to make them outcasts, they said, marked for death for dishonoring their families—especially hers.

Zakia has taken refuge in a women's shelter here. Even though she is legally an adult under Afghan law, the local court has ordered her returned to her family. "If they get hold of me," she said matter-of-factly, "they would kill me even before they get me home."

Neither can read, and they have never heard Shakespeare's tale of doomed love. But there are plenty of analogues in the stories they are both steeped in, and those, too, end tragically. . . .

"The story of true love in Afghanistan," said Reza Farzam, an Afghan university professor, "is the story of death."

CHAPTER 12

The Lovers

On March 9, 2014, I published a front-page story in the *Times* with the headline "2 Star-Crossed Afghans Cling to Love, Even at Risk of Death."

The story was about a young couple, eighteen-year-old Zakia and twenty-one-year-old Mohammad Ali, who are both Muslims but of different ethnicities and sects in Afghanistan. They had fallen completely, passionately, albeit chastely, in love. Their families were outraged, determined that they would never be together, and the threat of murdering them was not merely rhetorical, but a literal possibility. I wrote about how their relationship unfolded but also used the story to illustrate the appalling circumstances for young people there. Young women were essentially the prisoners of their families—objects and property, not free human beings. Illiterate, poor, and living in rural Afghanistan, the young couple attempted to do things the right way. Mohammad Ali went to her parents' home twice, begging for their daughter's hand in marriage. The second time, Zakia's brothers beat him so badly that he had to be hospitalized.

And yet, they persisted. Zakia eventually escaped from her family to seek protection in a women's shelter in another small city. But the court ordered her to return to her family, and when the shelter did not release Zakia, two women who worked in the Women's Ministry and had been advocating for Zakia were suspended.

The story turned out to be a sensation. *Times* readers' comments poured into the paper, expressing their support for the couple and offering money to help them get out of Afghanistan. The reaction from the American public and all over the world was something that I had never experienced in my entire career as a reporter. The paradox: no matter how remote the *New York Times* might seem in Afghanistan, by publishing the couple's story in that newspaper, I ended up exposing them to even more danger. Afghan media picked up the piece, and Zakia's and Mohammad Ali's portraits were published all over the place, further complicating their attempts to hide.

But even with this overwhelming attention, there was not much that could be done to improve their situation. Zakia was in the shelter, and the judges in the community were all on her family's side. As I thought about it then, I figured she would eventually be turned over to her family, and I'd be writing a follow-up piece about her being killed. But then she surprised me. Zakia escaped, met up with her beloved, and the two eloped. This, of course, made an even better story. Her escape was quite dramatic; a crowd of interested parties pursued her. I tried to track the couple down, a bit conspicuously— with my cameraman, translator, videographer, and fixer. Our presence in the search naturally increased the likelihood that they would be found by others, a depressing fact that did nothing to curb the intensity of our mission. We were racing to beat the police, as well as the couple's families. This contest had the highest of stakes—life or death, truly.

My team and I beat everyone else, but only by a few hours. Zakia and Mohammad Ali had traveled to a remote mountain area, where people hadn't laid eyes on a foreigner in years. When we found them, living with the few relatives who supported their decisions, they were broke and terrified, though also happy and triumphant, because they were now married.

If my team hadn't met them, if we hadn't been the ones to reach them first, they quite simply would not have survived. When we arrived, I saw how dire their situation was, and I made a decision that I have never regretted—but one that has caused me some grief and drawn a lot of criticism. For the first time in my decades-long career, I became part of the story. (It is strange to reflect on that fact now, because the second time that happened was when I wrote the piece about my brain tumor.) I gave the couple a substantial amount of money and put them in my car to help them escape. I wrote the story but kept my part in it a secret from my editors and the public.

On April 21, 2014, my story appeared—"Afghan Newlyweds, Facing Threats, Find Brief Respite in the Mountains." We had videos of Zakia and Mohammad Ali walking together, crossing a muddy stream, recounting their travels and fears of being arrested by the government. We showed the unforgiving landscape they had traveled and the mountainous region in which they hid. The reaction around the world was overwhelming once again. Activists demanded I do more than just write about them, and some wealthy readers reached out to me, offering financial support to help the young couple. I ended up working with some of those readers, once I stepped in to change the course of history and their fate. This young couple had little sense of how to cope with the world outside Afghanistan.

This was a unique case, and there was no question about what was right or wrong. No one—aside from a few mullahs and her family—would debate that having a young woman killed because she wanted to marry for love was morally wrong. But I was the kind of journalist who never even voted in presidential elections because I felt that I should not take partisan positions. For me, becoming involved like this was a radical decision, one rooted in morality, not journalistic standards. If Zakia had been picked up by the police in that remote region, I have no doubt that, over the three-hour drive to headquarters, the officers would have raped her before obeying the court order and returning her to her family—at which time she likely would have been murdered.

But naturally, in the weeks and months that followed, it all got a bit messier. Once aid was offered, how could it be withdrawn, or even limited?

Assistance came from unusual, even improbable sources. A man who referred to himself as "America's rabbi," the Orthodox rabbi Shmuley Boteach, who had a television show and had written over thirty books, dove into the case. He had read the story in the *Times* when it first appeared and then received a call from Miriam Adelson, the wife of the right-wing billionaire Sheldon Adelson, who was so touched by what I had written, she wanted to help. The two of them went on their own kind of *jihad*, meeting with anyone they could to persuade them to let the couple into the country. They met with Samantha Powers, then the American ambassador to the UN. Miriam Adelson's organization, The World Values Network, offered a generous grant and helped rescue the head of the Women's Ministry in Afghanistan, who had lost her job and been threatened because she had helped Zakia escape the family who had vowed to kill her.

Eventually, there were no more stories to write about this couple for the *Times*, so I proposed writing a book about them. After winning a bidding war among a dozen major US publishers, Harper-Collins published *The Lovers: Afghanistan's Romeo and Juliet, the True Story of How They Defied Their Families and Escaped an Honor Killing* in 2016. The book was translated into eleven languages and published in a dozen countries. Only after that book came out did things dramatically change for the young couple. An official high in the US government (I later learned who it was but was sworn to secrecy) read the book and was moved to arrange for the couple to be granted an unusual visa, known as humanitarian parole, allowing them to settle in America. At Rabbi Shmuley's urging, Miriam Adelson donated a significant amount of money to a refugee advocacy NGO in New Haven, Connecticut, which the agency used to get Zakia, Mohammad Ali, and their two young children into housing, also providing medical care and English lessons.

Years later, after my illness became public, my phone rang late one night, and to my surprise, it was Mohammad Ali, the Romeo, calling to wish me well. I was even more surprised that he spoke to me in pretty fluent English. It came as a bit of a shock since all our previous conversations had been mediated by a Farsi-English interpreter. The couple continued living in New Haven, where Mohammad worked as a handyman in rental properties as well as a driver for a dealer who needed cars delivered to various parts of the United States. Amazingly, his Afghan driving license was valid in the United States. Accustomed to the horrendous roads in Afghanistan, he found American expressways a pleasure to navigate.

When my book came out in 2016, Sheila and I had been separated for more than ten years.

When we first split up, we tried to keep our family together as best as we could. We had agreed that if my foreign posting changed, we would both have to agree on the new one and move together, if "together separately," meaning that we would maintain two households. That was feasible—just—since foreign correspondents always had company-provided housing where they were based. I would have to pay for only one place, while the company provided the family home. But maintaining two complete households for a family of five proved financially burdensome, despite the housing support. For instance, when I was hired by the *Times* to cover Iraq, in 2009, they initially posted me to Rome as my base, and Sheila and I both got places there, a couple of miles apart. We spent Christmases together, usually alternating one year with my family in Philadelphia and the next year with her family in England. By the time my career as a war correspondent really peaked, the kids were in their teens, and as the wars in Iraq and Afghanistan dragged on, into their college years and young adulthood. This is never an easy time for a family—parents can no longer tell their kids what to do, and the kids become adults, free to do as they choose, for good or bad. It was especially tough for a family like ours, with a mostly absent dad and an aggrieved mom. My many close friends were scattered around the world, so I had no real personal life in London or in Rome, except when my far-flung friends made the long trek to visit me in London (or I flew to see them, benefiting from millions of accumulated air miles).

I pour all my energies into journalism and work. From 2006 to 2016, I ran or helped run two war-zone news bureaus while also producing weekly, and later daily, and sometimes even award-winning news stories. *Newsweek* began publishing daily reports on its website in 2007, which helped prepare me for my return to daily journalism when the *New York Times* hired me in 2009 to cover Iraq. In my spare time, such as it was, I managed to write three full-length books, only one of which, *The Lovers*, has so far been published. I made peace with my circumstances and buried my loneliness in a rewarding mountain of work. So the last thing I was expecting, when I went to a TV studio in London early in 2016 to promote *The Lovers*, was to meet the love of my life: Leila Segal. We met in the TV studio's greenroom. She was also there to promote her first book, *Breathe*, a collection of short stories about Cuba, where she had been living the previous six years. Leila was also working at an NGO she had founded to help women who were victims of human trafficking. She was a poet—and quite beautiful. As we chatted before our respective television interviews, I knew that this was someone I wanted to see again. I didn't know it then but sensed, and would soon find out, that she was scary smart; she had finished secondary school—doing her A levels by age sixteen—two years before the norm. She completed a university law degree and law school, and passed the bar exam, in a total of four years. Of course, I googled her early on. Some people think doing so is a tad creepy, but how could I not? The first thing that came up was a picture of her wearing her white horsehair barrister's wig, just hiding her long, thick brown hair. Nearly six feet tall, she was my first romantic partner taller than I am. She was really someone I could look up to—and not just because of her height. As it turned out, she felt the same way. My opening line was to repeat my long-held complaint that the greenroom—the waiting room for guests appearing on TV—was not actually *green* in décor. I had been in many of them, since television appearances had long since become obligatory for foreign correspondents, especially ones who sometimes frequented interesting or hard-to-get-into places. Later, as all happy couples do, we spent hours turning our love's origin story over and over.

We both felt that, from the moment we met, we *saw, really saw* each other; isn't that what we're all looking for in a partner? To be seen, really seen by the other. We both sensed the deep hurt we each had at the core of our being—I from my turbulent childhood and a series of unhappy love affairs, she from a lifetime of feeling othered. We both felt that our childhoods were bruised by a feeling of being an outcast, each for very different reasons. And we both were still looking to heal that. We were both nesters at heart and our nests were pretty much empty. She was then forty-nine, and as beautiful as she had been at thirty. Early in our affair I found myself lamenting that we had not met when we were still young enough to have children together. Later she told me she felt the same way. In a text to me she said: "I realised that when I met you, I wanted both to heal you with my love and to shelter within yours."

I texted her back: "I have lots to say about that, Leila. I've long thought, and I think so have you, that we were drawn to each other at least in part because we sensed the same hurt in one another. And saw the other as both a refuge and a kindred soul.

"Only people who have lived trauma can understand it, that's why so many war vets refuse to talk about it to civilians."

Almost the first day after we became lovers, I hit the road, heading off to Afghanistan, where I was in my eighth consecutive year as a correspondent and bureau chief for the *Times*. Though we managed to speak by phone or text every day, that separation was one of many early trials our love affair had to endure. The biggest was my marital status and my doomed efforts to hold my family together. When Leila and I met in 2016, I had already been separated from Sheila for more than a decade; for the sake of family and my relationships with my children, I had not yet sought a divorce, and we often celebrated holidays together as a family. We even went on summer vacation together, to the beach house south of Rome that I had bought for the family many years before. Leila never asked me to get a divorce, but I was keenly aware that I was keeping her in the position of being in a relationship with a married man. And I was also well aware of the tired cliché: the man who says he's planning to divorce but never does. But she loved, trusted, and believed in me, which only made me love her more.

The biggest test was the terrible ordeal I put her through in our first summer, 2017, when I went for August holidays at my family's little beach house, Villa Mappa (after the many maps on the walls inside) with Sheila and our kids. In retrospect, it's astonishing that Leila continued to believe in me and in the possibility of us. I could see what it cost her and finally decided, all on my own, to file for divorce. Given how long Sheila and I had already been separated, Leila could hardly be considered "the other woman." But that didn't stop my children from reacting against her as such, at least at first, and for two years they hardly spoke to me and would not visit my home if Leila was there, which she often was.

Our relationship deepened. She traveled with me to Finland, Italy, Lithuania, and Iceland. My trip with her was the first time I'd ever visited Dixie (as the region's journalists call Israel, to guard against slipping and using the I-word, especially among Arabs) except as a war correspondent covering the first and second intifadas, the outbreaks of street and aerial warfare in Gaza and the West Bank, and Israel's invasions of Southern Lebanon.

In London she introduced me to that literary world from which I had always felt excluded as a journalist. We went on the road around Britain, attending literary festivals and events promoting our respective books, attending readings and dinners with friends, and reading our own and others' poetry at little joints in Soho. I was soon going to India to fill in for the *Times* bureau chief there, who was going on vacation for a month that summer. I loved working in India, where there are riveting stories wherever you turn, plus the *Times* had an impressive bureau there.

I suggested that Leila get a tourist visa and come along with me. We could go early and trek up to a hill town at the edge of the Himalayas. It was that season just before the onslaught of the southwest monsoon, when temperatures peak in the upper 120s Fahrenheit and humidity approaches 100 percent—weather we both loved and tolerated well, she from her years in rural, non-air-conditioned Cuba, I from my first foreign posting, in Bangkok, from 1978 to 1980.

Our time together there was perfect. And then she had to return to London, and I needed to get to work, and the bottom was about to fall out of our world.

PART II

After the Monsoon

"FROM HOTEL TO HOSPITAL: THE PERILS
OF REPORTING IN PAKISTAN"
New York Times
November 10, 2015

ISLAMABAD, Pakistan—The last time I worried about being the victim of a poison gas attack was in Baghdad, back when we still believed in the WMD fairy tale. The last place I ever expected a poison gas attack was in a five-star hotel here in Pakistan's capital.

That, however, is more or less what occurred Monday morning when I stepped into room 245 of the Marriott Hotel. I ended up in the hospital an hour later. . . .

Monday morning, the Marriott was being fumigated by the pest-control company, and it had apparently just sprayed the corridor on the second floor although not, the hotel management said, the rooms themselves; most, like mine, had their doors closed.

Some of the spray might have filtered through the gap at the bottom of the door, however, and I had turned off the air conditioning in my room.

The moment I stepped inside I started coughing but thought little of it since I had just gotten over a cold. The coughing grew worse and worse . . .

I called reception and asked if they would send a doctor, and they said he would be there in 15 minutes—five-star hotels, you would expect that—so I tried sitting down. I was also mysteriously sleepy between bouts of violent hacking, but going to sleep seemed like a bad idea because I was not really sure from where my next breath was coming. . . .

Then and there I decided I was never again going to stay in a hotel where the windows do not open, no matter how many stars it might have.

The Marriott's managers fessed up immediately to the ongoing fumigation and, at my insistence, agreed not to charge me for the night.

The American embassy helpfully directed me to one of the city's two best private hospitals, Kulsum International, nestled on the upper floors of an otherwise shabby-looking shopping mall, at least in part because there was a University of Chicago–trained pulmonologist there. The diagnosis: minor damage to the passages in my lungs, which was treated with corticosteroids and a nebulizer with the sort of medications used to relieve a severe asthma attack.

Sometime in the middle of the night, a couple of worried Marriott officials dropped by to share their condolences—and confusion. No one else in the hotel, it seems, succumbed to the gas. Was I perhaps allergic or asthmatic? Unfortunately for that theory, I am neither.

After they took their leave, I saw that the hotel officials had left what was the biggest gift basket of fruit I had ever seen. It could have fed an entire primary school, and since we have a policy at the *Times* of never accepting presents, I asked the hospital staff to give it to someone needy.

I could see the words "American" and "Lawsuit" taking shape in the Marriott officials' minds when they visited me at the hospital, especially after I refused their offer to return to the Marriott with an upgraded room. They need not worry. Life is too short to spend it in court, especially in Pakistan.

CHAPTER 13

The Middle Finger of God

After I was struck down by my first, and worst, seizure on the street in New Delhi on July 5, 2019, the first person to arrive by my hospital bedside was Leila, who could still travel with the tourist visa she had gotten for our very recent, and now unthinkably remote, holiday there. We had not included a hospital on our list of destinations, but it briefly became the center of our universe. We had only recently moved in together in London. On July 6, the very day after my seizure, Leila arrived and took charge of my treatment, keeping my employers, my family, and my friends informed of what was going on. Leila also had to help the nurses subdue me because I was trying, rather violently apparently, to climb out of my hospital bed. In the end they had to use leather-and-Velcro restraints, which I later realized were the source of bruises on my wrists and ankles, forearms and legs.

Naturally, I remember none of this but heard all about it later from Leila, who witnessed it while frantically calling friends, family, and colleagues, asking for help. At six feet in height, she's bigger than me but nowhere near as strong. The *Times* immediately hired a private male nurse to help her.

Once it is diagnosed, glioblastoma is considered a stage 4 cancer—meaning it is incurable. I titled my next journal "The Middle Finger of God," after I realized that I was afflicted with a disease with no known environmental or lifestyle causal factors. Even heavy smoking isn't associated with a greater risk of getting it—as it is with almost every other form of cancer. For me and for others, this invader of the brain can be attributed to only the cruel, capricious vagary of chance. Why on earth did I bother to eat all that kale? (A tombstone in a *New Yorker* cartoon put it that way.)

So, you get a dire diagnosis, and even if you are not a journalist, you start doing the research. But if you *are* a journalist, the intensity of that research is supercharged—you go deep, audaciously interviewing folks who might know more *so you can get to the bottom of the story*. I badgered my doctor friends for access to medical websites, which meant "find the best treatment, get the best doctors, cure the uncurable." And naturally, everyone you know—family, friends, fellow reporters—is doing the same thing. You start simply by googling "glioblastoma multiforme" and are assaulted by words like "incurable," "highly aggressive," "poor prognosis," "always fatal." You find the Glioblastoma Foundation. You see that the organization is "Transforming Glioblastoma Therapy." (And you wonder why it needs to be transformed.) And the answer appears: the foundation complains and lobbies for action to address the fact that the standard of care hasn't changed in forty years, nor have survival rates. "Glioblastoma is an aggressive and devastating cancer, with a median life expectancy for patients of 15 months post diagnosis. The long-term prognosis for glioblastoma remains poor. The current standard of care consisting of surgery, chemotherapy with Temodar, and radiation, is not very effective."

You discover that you are one of the approximately fifteen thousand Americans who are diagnosed with this wretched disease every year. And you also discover that men are 50 percent more likely than women to be diagnosed with glioblastoma. Well-educated white men get this cancer more than any other demographic, and the median age for those of us who are conscripted to fight in this war is sixty-five. You keep searching and find another brain tumor site that tells you that the five-year survival rate for glioblastoma patients is 7.2 percent. (It appears that things have marginally improved since my diagnosis, thus making my "6%" T-shirt obsolete.)

And then you start looking for the boldface names, the GBM-4 poster guys—now all dead—to see what they went through. John McCain was eighty and running for president when he was diagnosed; Ted Kennedy was seventy-six. Each lived only a year. Beau Biden was forty-one when his headaches, numbness, and paralysis landed him in the hospital—but he was diagnosed as having had a mild stroke. Then, in 2013, he joined our exclusive club, and two years later he was dead at forty-six. I got my news around my seventieth birthday. I cannot begin to figure out what this means in terms of the actuarial tables, but in terms of my life, there were already more yesterdays than tomorrows when glioblastoma reared its ugly head in July 2019, which was nearly three and a half years ago as I write this.

At first, it seemed as if the seizures, not to mention the tumor's assault on my brain, had come out of nowhere—in an instant. But when my memory rallied, I recalled that, for almost a year, I had been getting aberrant headaches every morning, very much like hangovers even though I wasn't drinking, and I am someone who very rarely suffers headaches. I blamed them on the statins I was taking due to high cholesterol. I had also experienced a somewhat weird rush of creative energy during this time, which was equally out of character. I am a hard-nosed, fact-based foreign correspondent with more than forty years' experience in war zones—a nonfiction guy through and through. But for unexplained reasons, and not only because of Leila's influence, I had begun writing poetry. I also took up—of all things—origami. Odder still, I even began making hand soaps. These new hobbies were pleasing and enjoyable, a yin to my life's yang, but where did they come from? They were at odds with my self-image as the rough-and-tumble war correspondent, the tough bureau chief managing staffs of dozens, in places like Kabul and Baghdad, Sarajevo and Kosovo, Skopje and Tirana. Stranger, perhaps, were the changes in my dispatches. They were more descriptive, more emotional; they had more brio. They were, in short, more "creative," if we understand the term to refer to that mysterious and liberating force behind works of imagination.

Could I point to all this as early evidence of a tumor beginning its incursion into my right parietal lobe—a region that manages the integration of one's five senses into language and cognition? And the place where, some scientists believe, creativity originates? Or is the answer as simple as this: I was in love with a poet. (Though that does not explain my headaches.) It is impossible for me to say.

Let me go over, once again, some of the facts recounted in my *New York Times* article that opened and has inspired this book. I was in New Delhi to cover for the bureau chief there. I was a couple weeks away from my seventieth birthday, and I went for a run, as usual ignoring and even reveling in the extreme heat. When I experienced the massive seizure on the street near a park, I was seen and saved by a Samaritan whose goodness is incalculable. I was unconscious and transported to a New Delhi hospital, where, once I regained something resembling consciousness, a physician told me my brain was now the home of a "space-occupying lesion." Repeating the next part of this anecdote is probably the whole point of my recounting the story again (although it does seem useful to set the scene): After doctors induced a coma to stop my seizures, the mortuary crew took me for dead and toe-tagged me with the following ID: "Unknown Caucasian male, age 47 and a half." Yes, years later, that story still gives me a twitch of pride and vanity, and makes me laugh a little manically. At first, I thought I might have been struck down by heatstroke, out jogging in 120-degree weather—and it was hardly dry heat. More like 90 percent humidity.

Leila, the first of my friends and loved ones to reach my hospital bed, supervised my move to Max Hospital, considered the best in New Delhi. She had no legal status in my life, even though she was the partner with whom I lived. But she managed to assert herself admirably and get things done on my behalf. Speed mattered. I needed aggressive care and treatment immediately, and my family, and friends, especially my close friend Matthew Naythons, MD, who also had my health-care mandate, faced the first of many crucial decisions: Should I return to the UK or be sent on a longer, and potentially dangerous, journey to the United States? Even in my impaired state, I was responsible for making the ultimate choice, and I finally agreed to be medevacked to New York City. I was headed to the Weill Cornell Medical Center, where my colleague Alissa Rubin had been successfully treated after her many injuries—including some serious head injuries—from the helicopter crash. It also happened to be one of the world's leading institutions in the treatment of glioblastoma.

The trip from Delhi to New York was remarkably comfortable, thanks to the generosity of the *Times*. Key to making this as safe as possible was Captain Catherine Scarr, a no-nonsense British army reserve officer and neurological nurse who proved impressively adept at getting a bag full of needles and scalpels through security checks during a few changes of planes. While not trained as a doctor, much less a surgeon, she had from time to time performed surgery over video links, with the surgeon using aircraft Wi-Fi. In Cathay Pacific's business-class cabin, much to the alarm of my fellow passengers, Captain Scarr strung up three sets of intravenous drips for me from the overhead bins—an antibiotic, a blood thinner, and a saline solution. My doctors had been worried about a heart attack or stroke from all the emboli swirling around in my system, hence Captain Scarr and her drips.

Further complicating matters was that we had embarked just as President Trump was threatening Iran with war, and airlines wouldn't risk traversing Iranian airspace. This meant we had to fly counterclockwise around the world, transforming a trip that would normally take twenty hours into forty. We went from Delhi, to Bangkok, to Thailand, to Hong Kong, and finally to New York. Whenever we changed planes, Captain Scarr would repeat the drill, marching through security with sharp objects, stringing up my drips, and remaining awake and alert to any changes, however small, in my condition. We were worried that I might not survive the journey, so I spent much of it rewriting my will and transmitting it to my lawyer over the plane's wonky Wi-Fi. I later learned that I had quite a few embolisms, a couple dozen in my lungs, several in two of my limbs, any of which could have easily migrated to the heart or the brain, with terminal consequences.

After finally arriving at Weill Cornell Medical Center to undergo the emergency brain surgery, I needed surgery because of those life-threatening embolisms. Captain Scarr reported that I had developed more embolisms en route, and she also suspected deep vein thrombosis, which was quickly confirmed in the ER. Because of the embolisms in my lungs and limbs, they installed a sub-vena cava filter—basically a fine screen to catch any errant emboli on the way from my lower extremities to my lungs, heart, or brain. Added to that, they found a hole in my heart between the right and left ventricles, once more heightening the risk that an embolism could exit that hole and reach an artery into my brain.

This delay of a few days turned out to be fortuitous, since is gave time for my friends, family, and colleagues from the *Times* to gather. I was gifted that glimpse into my Second Life, a vision of being surrounded by love. My once-estranged children, scattered in three different countries—Italy, Spain, and Britain—and their mother flew in to join me in the ICU. Brothers and sisters in Philadelphia appeared, with a couple of my nieces and nephews. Alissa was there—not only as a friend, but also as an informal independent patient advocate. Since my surgeon had operated on her, she knew what it meant to be a patient with a brain injury at that hospital. Matthew Naythons, my physician friend and partner in crime, appeared from California.

My first days in that hospital were plagued with seizures. The first and strongest I handled with the recitation of a memorized poem—a game Leila and I used to play. This time I was doing it to prove my brain was still working just fine, despite evidence to the contrary, such as my heavily slurred speech and a pronounced drool from the left side of my mouth.

Dr. Stieg's business card identified him as the hospital's "brain surgeon in chief," and this alpha male certainly dressed the part. A fashionista friend of mine opined that his Hermès tie probably cost a thousand dollars; I didn't know there was such a thing as a thousand-dollar necktie. Nurses half his age raved about how handsome he was. One evening in the ICU after the surgery, the curtain to my room had been pulled across the door to the corridor, leaving a twelve-inch gap at the bottom. There I could see a beautiful pair of shoes pausing just outside.

"Come in, Dr. Stieg," I called from my bed.

He then said, "How did you know it was me?"

"I don't know anyone else around here who wears three-hundred-dollar shoes."

With a tone of possibly mock offense, he replied, "These aren't three-hundred-dollar shoes, they're twelve-hundred-dollar ones."

Before my surgery, in addition to a barrage of scary statistics and prognoses, Dr. Stieg did deliver some good news. He had a tradition: whenever he operated on the birthday of a patient, he brought the person a cake prepared by the hospital's gourmet chef—the one they bring in for Saudi billionaire patients. I imagine the cost for that cake has disappeared somewhere in the hospital's $400,000 bill to date. I chose a chocolate mousse cake and had an impromptu birthday party with friends and family, including one Kabul colleague, Mujib Mashal, who flew in from his vacation in Paris for the occasion. "You did this all for the cake," someone joked.

Finally, on Wednesday, July 17, Dr. Stieg and his team cut out an area of bone from my skull and then delicately went in to excise a lime-sized mass of cancer from my right parietal lobe. They extracted 99.99 percent of the tumor, to slow its growth and address all the symptoms I was having. By Saturday, I was moved to the ICU stepdown unit and put in a lovely corner room, facing the East River. I described it as "an ICU with a view." And then more visitors appeared.

One night, I woke up at 4 a.m. and found my daughter Johanna, a photographer, perched on the edge of my bed. Together we looked at the many-windowed apartments on Roosevelt Island out in the East River; we talked about sketching the scene and how the focal point would be the huge real-estate sign facing the Upper East Side, reading "Space Available." It was a moment of special intimacy. I woke up later that morning to find her gone, but two pages of my journal were full of her sketch of that scene, done crookedly, with her left hand, she noted. I assumed she did this in solidarity with my left hand, impaired by the surgery (she is a righty, as am I). Next to the "Space Available" sign she put a little thought bubble with "brain metaphor?" written inside.

Another day after my surgery, I had a somewhat severe seizure, and immediately seven doctors appeared at my bedside. They were worried about bleeding in the tumor resection cavity, a common and life-threatening aftereffect of brain surgery. They immediately ordered an emergency CT scan of my brain, requiring that we rush down to the scanning theater. No one from the transport department was available though, so two of the doctors jumped on the back of my motorized bed to drive it themselves—a task well below their pay grade—rather than waste precious time waiting for someone else during a suspected brain bleed.

The poem I had been memorizing that day was Yeats's "Second Coming." As the docs sped us out of the room, I declaimed to Leila and the docs and anyone else who might be within earshot the line "Mere anarchy is loosed upon the world." Then, as the motorized bed gathered speed in the corridor, I called out, "The blood-dimmed tide is loosed upon the land," which I thought was a good line for a suspected brain bleed. Spurred on, they carried on racing through the corridors at high speed and taking the turns too tightly, so that on several occasions my poor bed bounced off the wall at a corner, all of which were well-padded and scarred from previous mishaps. "I hope you guys are better doctors than you are drivers," I observed. I was scanned, and the results were transmitted to Dr. Stieg, who immediately ordered a new course of treatment. Total elapsed time, from seizure to revised treatment plan, was under ten minutes.

In early August, I was released from the hospital to begin the next chapter of my new life. While in the hospital, I had jotted down some lines from the *Odes*, which the Latin poet Horace wrote in 23 BCE. "Better far to bear the future . . . like the past," he wrote. "Seize the present." This is the famous line, now a hardy Latin cliché, *carpe diem*. But then he finishes the poem with an even more profound, and certainly less well known, observation: "*Quam minimum credula postero.*" Which means "Trust tomorrow e'en as little as you may."

"ST. GEORGE'S AND THE TREE"
New York Times
October 26, 2009

BAGHDAD—Surrounded by glass and steel government buildings, some of them bombed-out shells from long ago, St. George's Church in downtown Baghdad has always seemed like something of an oasis.

Ever since the United States started using high explosives diplomacy with Iraq, the little Anglican church has had one close call after another.

Built in 1936 by the British military during their occupation of Iraq, the church lost some of its famous stained-glass windows when the United States military bombed a nearby building in 1992, and more were destroyed during the invasion in 2003, leaving only three examples remaining. They were mementos of British regiments stationed there.

Sunday the last three stained glass windows were blown out by the suicide bomb blasts that destroyed three Iraqi government buildings nearby, according to the church's lay pastor, Faiz Georges.

Once again, the church narrowly escaped disaster. Although the bombs went off at 10:30 a.m. on Sunday, church services and Sunday school weren't scheduled until afternoon and the church grounds were mostly deserted. Some 500 Iraqi Christians normally attend services there.

Many of the outbuildings were damaged, especially its charity clinic, and cars in the parking lot were incinerated, but none of the few people around were hit by flying glass or anything else. . . .

The church would have been much more heavily damaged, said Mr. Georges, if a windstorm had not blown a tree down on the road outside the night before. That forced the bomber to use the other side of the road. "It was a miracle," Mr. Georges said.

CHAPTER 14

My Brain, a User's Guide

I had taken my brain for granted these many years. Don't we all? I never appreciated its dazzling complexity, its resilience, its fragility, and, alas, its occasional unreliability. But there is nothing like a brain tumor to concentrate the mind, so to speak, even as it does its best to shred one's capacity to use it. Demonstrating, as it does, the profound differences and interdependence between our minds and our brains.

Now that nearly all of my space-occupying lesion had been evicted, I had to cope with the collateral damage it left behind. Part of that involved a complete loss of sensation on my left side, especially my left hand, which had as a result become nearly useless. Even for someone who is right-handed like me, this is inconvenient. My proprioception—the body's ability to figure out where it is in space without having to actually *think* about it—was utterly out of whack. I would walk into doors or bump into tables. Like some toddler learning to walk, I discovered that taking tumbles was part of my life—unlike a toddler, given the anticoagulating drugs I was taking, I could face dire consequences from a fall.

And then there were my seizures.

In an effort to prove to everyone—doctors, loved ones, but mostly myself—that my brain was OK, and to reduce the threat by laughing at it, I started giving often comical names to my seizures. Stranger still was that, in an odd way, I even started to look forward to them. Almost any sort of stress or excitement would set one off, but the ones post-surgery were different from the extravagantly physical, flailing variety of the grand mal one I had in India, before I was operated on, when my brain tumor first expressed itself seriously. Eventually, the only physical manifestation of my seizures was slurred speech and a left-side drool. But even such mental seizures (called "focal seizures" by neurologists) were a big concern to doctors because they could sometimes lead to a stroke and even death.

Seizures are basically an unusual burst of electricity in the brain that can last from a few seconds to several minutes. These bursts can start in one spot and reverberate, disrupting thoughts, memories, movement, nearly all parts of one's functioning. When I was still in the hospital and seemed to be acting a little strange, as though I might be having a seizure, I was subjected to what they called the smile test. This is a basic neurological exam to determine if a patient has had a seizure. A neurologist tells the patient to smile and then checks the symmetry of the smile. If that doesn't look right, it's time for the patient to stick their tongue out at the doctor, which can seem odd. But a tongue hanging out is even more subject to asymmetry and a reliable way to see whether a seizure is taking place. With my daughter Johanna's help, we constructed a smile mobile at home, using pictures of my smile, along with other random smiles. And with some unused brain drains as counterweights. We were both bemused to discover that a brain drain was an actual piece of medical equipment used to collect excess fluids during surgery, and not just a geopolitical metaphor.

For a while after brain surgery, nearly anything could set off a seizure. Talking with my son, Jake, about playing squash, I told him about how in Kabul we had a homemade court that a few of us used regularly. It had a leaking roof and often puddles, which were dangerous, since in squash you move fast, changing direction frequently and suddenly. The last thing you want is to slip in a puddle, so we adopted the practice of calling "wets" in addition to calling "lets." A let in squash is what a player calls when another player is caught between him and the ball, blocking his stroke, so the point gets replayed; if a puddle was between the player and the ball, we added a rule that we could call a "wet" and replay the point. During this conversation with Jake, we both started laughing so hard, it set off another seizure—the "Squash Wets" seizure.

Doctors, determined to control my seizures, administered an anti-seizure drug known as Keppra. My brain both loved and loathed Keppra. It calmed my seizures to be sure; it also unleashed anger that I would have much preferred to repress. Doctors later explained that Keppra was well known for causing a phenomenon dubbed "Keppra rage"—which, for a man who had harbored a great deal of anger for a great deal of his life, was *not* a good thing. The drug's official list of side effects uses anodyne words like "irritability," "mood swings," and "disinhibition." Keppra brought out the worst in me. But, as the oncologist explained, it was one of the few anti-seizure meds available that would not interfere with the chemotherapy drugs they were likely to use on me.

If this elixir was going to allow me to have the chemotherapy that would save my life, I rationalized, enduring a bit of bad temper was not too high a price for those around me to pay. As it turned out, I had no idea that, indeed, it was an extremely high price to pay, perhaps too high. Especially for Leila, who, being the person closest to me and around me the most, naturally got the worst of it.

During my Keppra period, I railed against her, telling her she should just leave me and forget about our relationship. I insisted that she was only making things worse by being around—all accusations that could not have been further from the truth. Although intellectually we both knew that this was the drug speaking, not the man who loved her, words matter and lodge in one's psyche, difficult, if not impossible, to banish. I inflicted horrible pain on her. I felt as if another being had taken over my mind, and especially my mouth. She was not the only person who experienced the firehose of my toxic emotions. But it all revealed how vulnerable our brains are to any changes in their chemistry. I nearly punched an unwelcome visitor to my ICU room, but fortunately my old friend Matthew, an ex-boxer himself, saw it coming (serious punches begin in the legs, which start to coil, are carried through the large muscles of the thighs and trunk, and only end in the arm and fist). He quickly restrained my right arm and hurried the visitor out.

Outside the hospital but still under Keppra's influence, I got into a shouting match with a city cop. My daughter Johanna heard about it and scolded me: "Dad, you always told us, never get in an argument with a cop, you're only going to lose. And never fight with a man with a gun. You broke both those rules." I was chagrined at being reminded of that but proud of her for remembering it.

As I mentioned, my tumor was located on my right parietal lobe, which is quite near the center of the brain, close to the back and top of the head. It's nestled behind the frontal lobe, which one might consider the air traffic controller of our lives—prioritizing, managing various functions, making sure that we do not blurt out the first thing that comes to mind. There are two parietal lobes, on the left and the right hemispheres of the brain, and as a very user-friendly website, Simply Psychology, informed me, they are "particularly important in integrating information from the body's senses to allow us to build a coherent picture of the world around us." In describing the key roles of the two sides of our parietal lobes, it notes, "The left side is believed to be important in keeping track of the location of parts of the body which are moving. The right side, however, is believed to be important in helping us keep track of the space around us."

Naturally, with an illness as aggressive as GBM-4, I needed radiation and chemotherapy to insure that the 0.1 percent of the tumor that Dr. Stieg left behind would not flourish and colonize new parts of my brain. Unlike many cancers—prostate, for instance, and some kinds of breast cancer—GBM is a "primary tumor," meaning not a metastasis from cancer elsewhere in the body, and it also does *not* metastasize to other parts of the body. Sounds positive, but in fact, this isn't good news. GBM's opportunism and eagerness to take over a brain is fatal and horrifying enough. The protocol was two weeks of radiotherapy around the area of the tumor, to get any cells that the surgery had missed, followed by treatment with chemotherapy using a drug called Temodar—which, thankfully, I seem to tolerate pretty well. I had eight sessions of chemo, in five-day rotations, for seven months. I took a tablet in the morning and another tablet to keep me from vomiting, and that was it. I didn't have to have infusions, as so many other cancer patients do. Radiation made me lose a bit of hair on the right side, but it grew back promptly. I have not suffered from debilitating nausea, a usual horror of chemotherapy. But adding this new ingredient to the existing assault on my brain from the seizures and surgery has resulted in a serious case of "chemo brain." Should Temodar stop working, and new glioblastomas develop, then my doctors will go into the toolbox for the really exotic treatments; these range from immunotherapy to gene therapy.

The tumor, the surgery, the radiation, and the chemotherapy amounted to a massive assault on my right parietal lobe, as well as neighboring brain tissues. I was shocked at how difficult the simplest aspects of life had become—putting on my shirt, buttoning a jacket, managing to loop a belt around my diminished waistline. I thought that part of my clumsiness and difficulty stemmed from chemo brain. I was predictably tired during my radiation treatment, but for me, chemo brain was probably the most vexing of the effects of my tumor. I would routinely forget basic things like the name of the month, the day of the week, the year, and whether I had taken my meds just three minutes earlier, when I actually had. It was a classic case of chemo brain with short-term memory loss, general forgetfulness, confusion, and occasional befuddlement. It's just a magnification of things that occasionally happen to all of us, even those who do not have brain tumors.

I'm one of the lucky GBM patients because I have what's known as a methylated gene, which means that I can tolerate large doses of chemotherapy and handle it for a longer period of time. But it becomes quite challenging to determine whether a certain level of dysfunction is because of chemo or because of the damage to my right parietal lobe. It often takes a couple years for the effects of chemo to completely wear off. My "chemo brain" counselor assures me that the level of disorientation I've experienced can sometimes last for two years before one's brain returns to normal and stops forgetting how to put on a belt.

But frequently I find myself putting my pants on backward, or even inside-out—or sometimes backward and inside-out. I'd put them on upside-down if I could, but apparently that cannot be done (yes, I have tested the theory). I'd often put my shirts on inside-out, and once I buttoned my outer jacket to my inner shirt in such a way that I couldn't open the jacket. I must assert that I've been dressing myself successfully for seven decades. But as it turns out, these are all *classic* problems that emerge from damage to the right parietal lobe, which is the part of the brain responsible for many self-care skills, like, say, getting dressed.

There is an astonishing range of traditional and cutting-edge new treatments that doctors plan to employ to beat back my tumor, should it recur or spawn new ones, which is, unfortunately, routine with GBM. For instance, Dr. Howard Fine, my neuro-oncologist, explained that they would sequence my entire genome and also the genome of the tumor, looking for mutations that might correspond to ones seen in other cancers. Then they would find the precise, most effective chemotherapy.

Another option, which fascinated me, was to extract stem cells from my brain and my tumor (which is preserved somewhere in a petri dish, probably). Placed in a hospitable environment, these stem cells could grow robust little baby brains, technically called "embryonic stem cell–derived organoids." These are actual tiny brains, identical to my own, DNA-wise, with neurons that fire electrical impulses. They could be bombarded with a host of potential chemotherapies, in order to see which would be most effective in stopping a tumor's growth, and I would then receive that treatment, should I suffer a recurrence or spread of the glioblastoma tumor. In short, doctors would practice killing the tumors in my "baby brains."

These medical interventions would be deployed only if my glioblastoma showed any sign of recurrence or spread. But so far, for reasons mysterious to me and my doctors, I have experienced none.

A raft of therapies—psychological, physical, occupational—helps me manage in the world. I have one physical therapist whose entire focus is on the hands, these essential, complex, and elegant appendages responsible for getting food to our mouths, clothes on our backs, keys into locks, and stories typed. When the part of the brain that makes these things second nature becomes damaged, these therapies can do an end run around that part of the brain and create new pathways elsewhere. That has been the case with my nearly useless left hand; I have had to relearn how to use it based on visual control rather than touch sensation. It's astonishing how many of our daily interactions with the physical world require two hands—especially those inventions of the devil, buttons.

Two years post-surgery, I finally could button my trousers as well as my shirt. Tie my shoelaces, knot a necktie. This may not sound like much, but being unable to button your shirt is both impractical and, if you have to ask someone else to do it for you, humiliating.

It makes you feel as if you're not a whole, independent person. For months and months, I worked on relearning this. When I finally did, it seemed a major achievement. Putting on gloves posed a different problem; I can now put on my left-hand glove more easily than the one for my right hand. My right hand still uses sensation to find where the fingers are inserted, but it doesn't always get things right. To put on my left glove, I use vision, as I've been trained to do by my hand therapist, and it has worked. When I was able to put on both gloves once more, I felt an almost giddy sense of accomplishment.

These experiences remind me of what it was like to be in high school, and studying, say, English with Miss Jenkins. When I wrote something that pleased her, and she rewarded me with praise, there was no feeling quite like it. It also was one that I never imagined enjoying as an adult, but then I started working with my brilliant hand therapist, and every time I reached some benchmark—a button buttoned, a belt buckled—I felt the same kind of almost child-like gratification at her praise.

One of my now-extinguished former points of pride was my impressive typing speed. With so much to express, I felt frustrated at having to record myself and have the words transcribed, or having to laboriously work in longhand with my fully functional right hand, as nearly all this book was written. So, my therapist gave me homework to try to get my brain understanding what it was like to type once again, summoning up old neural pathways. For this, I used the latex dust cover for my computer keyboard from my work in very dusty war zones like those in Iraq. It fit over each key quite snugly, so it protected them while I typed. I unearthed this dust cover, put it in my lap, and used my fingers to go over the keys, reacquainting them with what it was like to type. Emily, the therapist, called it air typing, meant to reawaken old neural pathways—what we often call "muscle memory" is actually brain memory.

When my kids were visiting me, we would play a game in which I would type in the air—and they would try to decipher what I was typing. It was not easy, for obvious reasons, until I did one of those sentences, cherished by typing instructors throughout the English-speaking world, that includes every letter of the alphabet, such as "The quick brown fox jumps over the lazy yellow dog." (There's a word for these sentences, which of course I've forgotten.) My son, Jake, who is a gamer and types at lightning speed, sometimes figured out what I was air typing. He clocks in at 125 words per minute compared to my previous best of 100; his sisters type in the low hundreds.

In addition to my hand therapist, my team includes a psychotherapist, a physical therapist for my back and walking, an occupational therapist, a chemo brain psychotherapist, and a neuropsychologist. My numerous neurologists include one who specializes in seizures, another in strokes, another who is an expert on memory. In case they need to radiate my brain again, I have a radiation oncologist. An Italian named Silvia Formenti, she has been talked about in the profession as a candidate for the Nobel Prize in medicine for her pioneering work in precisely targeting radiation, almost down to the cellular level, thereby minimizing the terrible side effects of radiotherapy, especially to the brain. I have doctors in specialties I never knew existed, like my neuro-ophthalmologist.

My weeks are consumed with appointments. My MRI brain scans were initially scheduled once every two months, standard for GBM patients, usually for the rest of their lives—a sword of Damocles hanging over our necks; this famously aggressive disease can return at any time, even after five years without a recurrence, which is considered for many cancers to mean the disease is effectively cured. Now, after so many clear scans, I get them only three or four times a year, followed by visits to my neuro-oncologist, Dr. Howard

Fine—the generalissimo among this corps of medical providers. Dr. Fine is a scientist as well as clinician, the lead researcher into GBM treatment at the National Institutes of Health. He says he has treated thousands of GBM patients. He chairs my tumor boards— I've never attended one of these meetings (I don't think patients are invited) but have heard about them—a convocation of the many doctors involved in the care of a brain tumor patient.

Now I see my medical care as my full-time job, and approach it very much like covering a war: the hospitals and clinics are my war zone, the surgeons and oncologists the generals and colonels, the technicians and nurses and the physical and occupational and psychotherapists the foot soldiers. I've made it my business to re-member the first name of every one of them, from the receptionists to the radiologists, much as I used to do with the soldiers, from the lowest private to the generals; they were all my protectors in the war zones where I've worked.

The enemy now, of course, is a microscopic bit of alien proto-plasm, cells numbering in the millions or even in single digits, lurk-ing, looking for an opportunity to multiply and spread—in the case of glioblastoma, via tentacles that snake through the brain and seed new tumors, which eventually, and usually, kill the patient. I no lon-ger get chemo—the damage that it does to the body now outweighs any benefits from further treatment. So now my only treatment is the keto diet, a healthy lifestyle, and a cheerful, irrepressible opti-mism, which many of my docs have assured me is the best thing I have going for me. I've faced that brain-scan sword of Damocles sev-enteen or eighteen times now, never doubting that the results would be clear.

Bleeding in the brain remains a big concern; it can be fatal, necessitating an emergency CT scan after any serious blow to the head. My daughter Lorine jokingly suggested that I was taking hits to the head deliberately to get brain scans ahead of schedule—I wasn't, of course, but the idea immediately crossed my mind when I found myself on the floor of the bathroom, after falling and hitting the front of my head on the edge of the bathtub so hard that I had a dramatic black eye, which took a couple of weeks to disappear.

My original prognosis in July 2019 was a median life expectancy of fifteen months. Thirty-eight months later, as of this writing, I'm still going strong. I've lost fifty pounds and six inches off my waist, thanks to the keto diet. My nutritionist has prescribed an intake of only forty-two grams of carbs a day—less than two small crackers, or possibly one piece of toast. But one is never hungry; the diet allows for all the fat and protein one wants. It has been demonstrated that ketones—which a high-fat diet forces the body to produce in place of glucose—effectively kill off cancer cells because they can't metabolize them. But the keto diet remains to be proven clinically with real GBM patients; I'm hopefully on my way to being the living proof of this.

Has all this increased my chances of surviving? Or is it just a matter of luck? Perhaps a combination of both. But so far, my terminator has failed to live up to its reputation. And I'm nearly a year and a half past my predicted survival. As an old friend said recently: for more than a year, old pal, you've been playing with the house's money. As a once inveterate casino gambler, I appreciated the joke.

"GHOSTS ON THE FRONT"
New York Times
August 31, 2009

FORWARD OPERATING BASE WARHORSE—Soldiers believe in ghosts. I know this because when I am with soldiers, it is the only time I believe in ghosts. Not surprisingly, soldiers never talk about this for fear of sounding foolish. Instead, they invest their surroundings with memorials and mementos.

They name their DFACs (Dining Facilities, once mess halls), their MWRs (Morale, Welfare and Recreation centers, or gyms), and any other semipermanent structures after the fallen. Even the roads in the big forward operating bases, like this one outside Baquba, in Diyala Province, sometimes take on the names of ghosts. Camp Warhorse, for example, named its Faulkenburg Theater after Command Sgt. Maj. Steven W. Faulkenburg, who died fighting in Falluja in November 2004.

The ghosts of the dead become a reassuring presence, so that the living know they themselves won't be forgotten.

CHAPTER 15

I Forget the Name of This Chapter: On Memory

Have you ever spent an hour looking for your glasses until someone pointed out to you that they were on your face? Have you ever lost your keys and spent a week looking for them, only to find them still in the door lock outside, for anyone to turn, or even in the car's ignition? Have you ever forgotten your best friend's wife's name briefly or struggled to find a word that you know you know very well? These sorts of things happen to me almost daily and are extremely vexing, but as I often say to people—you've done things like that too, right? And when they confirm they have, I pounce good-naturedly: "But then I have a malignant brain tumor. What is your excuse?"

Often, it's just age. It doesn't have to be a brain injury like the glioblastoma multiforme stage 4 that I have. It doesn't mean that you're getting Alzheimer's disease, but it is a problem that a lot of us have as we get older, and the good news is that there is something you can do about it. It's not taking one of those weird drugs like Prevagen (made from a jellyfish protein that glows in the dark) advertised on late-night television in commercials that spend more time listing all the terrifying possible side effects than the promised benefits. No scientific studies have shown any benefit to memory or the brain from taking nootropic supplements, as these supposed brain-enhancing compounds are called. Dr. Phil Stieg, chairman of the neurology department at Weill Cornell, called the nootropics unproven and useless. Part of the problem is that they're usually sold—at high cost—as nutritional supplements over the counter and thus do not undergo the rigorous testing required for prescription drugs. The Federal Trade Commission has outright called Prevagen, the most heavily marketed nootropic, a "hoax." And New York state brought a lawsuit, along with the FTC, against Prevagen's marketer, Quincy Bioscience LLC, seeking to prevent the use of unproven claims to market and sell Prevagen and asking the courts to force the return of profits earned from the supplement. New York's attorney general, Eric Schneiderman, said, "The marketing for Prevagen is a clear-cut fraud, from the label on the bottle to the ads airing across the country." He stated that the company's own internal studies show that it does not work.

While there is probably no magic pill to help fix our fading recollections, there is still plenty that people can do to exercise their brain, memory experts say. It's all about using the natural neuroplasticity of the brain to create new neural pathways that compensate for deficits. This is becoming a significant issue as the seventy-five million baby boomers reach their sixties and seventies, and they're all losing their keys, forgetting their passwords, and looking for their glasses until they find them, right on their reddening face.

I had a particular personal interest in improving memory because of the multiple traumas to my brain, from my brain tumor itself, the surgery to remove it, seizures, debilitating treatments including chemotherapy, radiotherapy, and so on. So I hunted for a neurologist who specializes in memory. And then I found one. Of course, I forgot his name almost immediately. But his name was unusual enough for me to manage to find him in a list of other neurologists: Dr. Makoto Ishii. And just how many people are concerned about memory issues was vividly demonstrated by how difficult it is to get an appointment to see Dr. Ishii. He seemed to be booked until the next century. After all, there are a lot of us baby boomers. Somehow I finally got an appointment, and he had a lot of practical advice for people worried about their memory. In my case, the traumas to my brain had reduced the size of my hippocampus, which is where neuroscientists believe short-term memories are made and stored. That was the bad news. "But the good news is," the doctor said, "there are things we can do about it," thanks to the neuroplasticity of the brain. We can retrain it.

Dr. Ishii had a ready list of things that can help. Play a lot of difficult games like chess, do crossword puzzles and sudoku, and the like. Learn a new language, learn to play an instrument, or just play more difficult pieces on the instrument you already play. Interestingly, Dr. Ishii didn't think that reading books would have much effect one way or the other since for most or many of us, it's something we all do pretty routinely, and usually passively, to educate, inform, or amuse ourselves, but not to stretch our brains. Much better to read books as part of a book club and to discuss them with a group of intelligent strangers. Those conversations alone, Dr. Ishii said, are good exercise for the brain and memory. Find people we're not used to talking to, people other than our partners or close friends. Find things that "take us out of our comfort zones," Dr. Ishii said. So, take up drawing or painting—but especially with another person, whether in the same space or on Zoom.

Dr. Phil Stieg says that the best thing you can do for your brain is to follow a healthy diet and get plenty of exercise, especially cardiovascular exercise. Dr. Richard Isaacson, who directs the Alzheimer's prevention project at NewYork-Presbyterian Hospital, put it more bluntly: "As the belly size gets larger, the memory centers get smaller." Dr. Stieg and Dr. Isaacson both recommend the DASH diet, which stands for "dietary approaches to stop hypertension." The DASH diet is recommended for people with heart disease, or people who want to prevent heart disease; essentially, it is the Mediterranean diet, low in salt, carbohydrates, and sugars. In Dr. Stieg's view, "A diet that's heart-healthy is also going to be brain-healthy."

In addition, good sleep hygiene and reduction of stress, particularly through meditation and mindfulness training, are important. Many doctors recommend these practices because of their scientifically proven usefulness in stress reduction. "Sleep itself, which gives the brain a chance to rest, has been proven scientifically to help improve brain health and memory," Dr. Ishii, the memory neurologist, said.

The standard screening exam given to patients with suspected neurological or cognitive disorders includes basic questions like these: What is the date and day of the week? The year? The address of the office where the exam is taking place? The name of the current president of the United States? During Trump's term in office, that was, sadly, an easy one to remember. Neurologists also frequently give a subject three random, unrelated words and tell them that they'll be asked later on to recall them. The first time I did that exam, I got two out of three, which is about average, apparently. But then I saw a clip of Donald Trump during a campaign appearance, responding to criticism of his intelligence. He boasted that he had been given this standard cognitive exam and was able to remember the three words perfectly, which he cited as proof of high intelligence. "Hardly anyone can get all three," he boasted. Yet another falsehood from that font of falsehoods.

I personally took that test result as a motivator. And motivation is certainly a big factor in working to improve memory. Determination works even better, in my experience. So, in future iterations of that exam, I tried hard to remember all three words, making up a sentence including them all—if someone as thick as Donald Trump can get all three words right, I knew I could do so too, and did. On one occasion the neurology nurse went off to do something else and forgot to return to ask me the three words. So half an hour later, I went to her office and sent a message in through the secretaries with the three words that she had forgotten to ask me: *purple, loyalty, elephant.* I'm pretty sure I got them all right.

Dr. Isaacson, one of the foremost experts on prevention of Alzheimer's disease, often works with people whose families have included many individuals diagnosed with Alzheimer's, and they fear they may well inherit it, since it's well-established that the genetic component of that disease is significant.

So he puts those people on the DASH diet or something similar and encourages them to improve their sleep hygiene and level of exercise and to reduce their stress and their consumption of carbs, sugar, and sodium. The goal is to prevent or delay the onset of Alzheimer's. "There are things one can do to prevent cognitive decline," Dr. Isaacson said.

Most people have problems with short-term memory. One can have terrible short-term memory problems but still have excellent recall for events that happened decades earlier, a phenomenon familiar to most older people and one for which I am personally quite grateful while writing this memoir of my forty years as a war correspondent. Long-term memory has proved invaluable and surprisingly good, considering that I lose track of my cell phone three or four times a day, or make that six or eight, since I usually carry at least two phones.

Memory is a funny thing. I'll forget a password I use every day and sometimes the date and time of an appointment that I had just made minutes before, but I can often remember in detail certain things from decades ago. One fine morning recently, completely out of the blue, I remembered the combination to the padlock I had used on my high school locker more than fifty years ago. It was a Master combination dial padlock: two times past 0 to the left to 26, and then back past 26 the opposite way to 12, then back past 12 to 6. Now I can't forget that piece of entirely useless information—that padlock disappeared decades ago—as much as I have tried to do so, feeling that it is just a complete waste of neurons, like an earworm of some song you don't even like. Those neurons could be put to better use remembering my Gmail password. But it doesn't work that way, sadly.

Short-term memory loss is often one aspect of chemo brain, along with the inability to perform some executive functions, such as scheduling. I need help keeping my calendar—and I often have trouble with basic arithmetic: addition, subtraction, and multiplication. Yet strangely, I can still work out quadratic equations from my college calculus course.

I often joke with people, "Have I told you about my short-term memory problems?" and then I make a laugh line out of it, repeating a little later, "Have I told you about my short-term memory problems?"

Or I just add this: "I forget."

"EVER WONDER WHAT IRAQIS FIND FUNNY?"
Newsweek
March 12, 2007

BAGHDAD—Even in its darkest days, Iraq has proven to be a target-rich environment for its jokesters. Saddam Hussein made a particularly good foil. When the former dictator was hung, goes one of recent vintage, the executioners asked him if he had any last requests. "Yes," he replied. "Call out the reserves!" (Iraqi reservists were called up repeatedly, some serving 20 years or more during his many wars.) Iraqis don't have Saddam to kick around anymore, but there's no shortage of replacement subjects. The jokes they tell now are not always terribly funny, at least to foreign ears, but they have a lot to say about their present predicament.

A lot of them are about fleeing the country, as 3.9 million have done already. Question: What's the best job in the Iraqi government? Answer: Foreign ambassador. Or: An Iraqi finds Aladdin's lamp and rubs it 'til the genie comes out. "Master, your wish is my command." The Iraqi asks him to make a bridge connecting Iraq to Europe, so he can run away. "Master, that is a very hard thing to do." Okay, the Iraqi tells him, then just make the situation in Iraq better. The genie thinks for a moment and replies, "How big do you want the bridge?" . . .

In a place best-suited now to black humor, the laughs come easily.

CHAPTER 16

This Is Not a Joke?

I have laughed my way through this disease, and while it may not compete with cutting-edge chemotherapies and a massive therapeutic support system, I've found it to be rather powerful medicine. "How are you?" people ask, concerned and a bit tentative. "I feel great," I reply cheerfully, "aside from the fact that I have terminal cancer." Leila has said that I need to ease up on the mordant humor. It upsets people, she observes. But being able to laugh at one's disease is empowering. And if I'm able to make a joke out of my cancer, well, so much the better. And truly, I have been feeling healthier than probably at any other point in my life—no longer drinking and now working out in the gym, taking long daily walks, sleeping well. All those benchmarks of health? Check, check, and check. Aside from having had a malignant brain tumor, I've been in great shape.

True, terminal cancer is no laughing matter, but that just makes the funny parts even more humorous. Where does that confidence come from? I'm tempted to say it's an attitude born from an innate appetite for danger, hardship, and conflict—and for staring them down.

Leila was not the only person who suggested that my rosy view might not comport with the realities I was facing. I attended a GBM patients' support group, back in the pre-COVID days when such things were possible. Once more, I would bring what I considered to be wit and charm to a gloomy gathering. There we sat, some of us with our partners, some hollow-eyed and desperate, others in the earlier stages, looking around with barely concealed horror at images of their future selves. How can you make a joke out of something so terrible as a life-threatening disease? Well, it's a matter of life and death for me too. What's the point of having a brain tumor if you can't act out with it?

As we sat together, I told a few jokes and recounted some of the things that had made me laugh since the beginning of my disease. I had the whole group laughing along with me before it was over, as I recounted my reaction to being put on hold by call-center operators as they embark on their insincere effort at friendliness.

"How are you today, Mr. Nordland?" they ask chirpily. "Do you mind if I put you on a brief hold?"

To which I reply, "Actually I do mind. I have terminal cancer and don't really want to spend what little time I have left listening to bad hold music. Can you just put me right through?"

Soon, I saw smiles on my fellow patients' faces.

We all suffered the indignities of chemo brain, which was further amplified by the fact that our brains were already under assault by tumors. I shared a story about the "contagion" of chemo brain. When a home health aide assigned to me went off to empty the garbage, she put the garbage bag in the refrigerator instead of the bin. "See," I said, "I told you chemo brain's contagious."

I used to love Pachelbel's Canon in D, but so many doctor's offices use it for hold music that I've come to despise that precious melody. And if a secretary for one of my twenty-four doctors offers me an appointment date a week in advance, I point out, "Hey, I have terminal cancer and I'm not sure I'll live that long."

"I'm the one with the brain tumor," I often say, which is often a real conversation stopper or argument topper. Even that line, given the right context, can be funny. It is also an act of defiance: maybe you will kill me, GBM, but you can't stop me from laughing at you.

One day I went to the Brain Tumor Center at Weill Cornell and the office of the neuro-oncologist Dr. Howard Fine. He is the founding director of the center and has been in charge of my post-surgical treatment. I was there that day because I had a profuse nosebleed. This was a serious concern because I was taking blood thinners to protect against pulmonary embolisms, and a nosebleed could suggest that I was too decoagulated, a state that could lead to other complications such as a bleed in my fragile brain. I was telling jokes to the women at the front desk and somehow the issue of Dr. Fine's sense of humor, or lack of it, came up. I said I could guarantee them that I could make him laugh.

They were skeptical. "You'll never get a laugh out of Dr. Fine," one of them said.

To be fair, I can understand their skepticism. The first thing that one thinks of when Dr. Fine comes to mind is that he is doing one of the most difficult, thankless, relentless jobs in medicine—and therefore in all the professions. He has devoted his life to caring for and doing research on behalf of patients with brain and spinal cord tumors, the sickest of the sick. Nearly all of us will die on his watch, no matter how much he manages to forestall the inevitable. He's been doing this for nearly thirty years and has treated more than twenty thousand patients. So, yes, not a field that inspires lots of fun and hilarity.

And yet . . . I had guaranteed I could break his reserve.

When Dr. Fine saw me, he noted that nosebleeds were a prob-lem that long predated my cancer, a testament to how well he knew my medical history down to the tiniest detail. I was impressed, but no less resolved to win my bet. "Did I ever tell you about the time I had a nosebleed as I was crossing the land border into Iraq?" I asked. "The nosebleed was so bad that it splattered my white shirt quite dramatically and also ran down onto my trousers, and there was blood everywhere, boxes of tissues could not stop the flow, and my face was bloody as well. I thought that looking like this was likely to present a problem getting into Iraq.

"When I got to the border checkpoint, the soldiers there scarcely showed any surprise or alarm at my condition. One of them even joked, 'Looks like he's seen Achmed already.' Achmed was the Mukhabarat officer at that checkpoint, an officer of the secret police notorious for roughing up visitors. Since I was already well bloodied, it seemed there was no need to detain me further, so the border guards stamped my passport and visas."

Even Dr. Fine started laughing at that anecdote, and I exchanged a triumphant glance with the receptionists.

In my new life, humor is not restricted to clever anecdotes, slightly old jokes, or snappy one-liners. Sometimes the situations I find myself in, given the addled state of my chemo-brained right parietal lobe, would not be out of place on a sitcom. Once Joe Kahn, the managing editor of the *New York Times*, visited me in the small apartment I have near Times Square, generously provided by our employer. I have known Joe for many years, and we had lots of contact during his earlier stint as foreign editor, when I was a lowly foreign correspondent on many troubled far shores. Joe may appear a bit remote and businesslike, but I have found that behind his reserved demeanor, he has a big, warm heart and a great sense of humor. Not to mention the fact that he is a terrific journalist.

When Joe arrived, I set up one of my folding camp chairs that I reserve for special guests, which spared us the awkwardness of sharing the loveseat sofa. As he sat in the chair of honor, I stood next to him talking, clearly unaware of the fact that I had put my trousers on backward—and without a belt around my now much slimmer waist.

As I stood there, holding forth about one thing or another, my pants simply dropped to my ankles. "Thank god I wore underwear today," I said, hoping to ease the embarrassing moment with a joke. "That's probably already more information than you need." Laughter filled the small apartment.

I have discovered truly wonderful dividends from my brain tumor, including a renewed family life and the multiple expressions of love from family and friends. But Leila and I were just beginning a new life together, and our future had been abruptly ripped away from us—in my case by my likely death, in her case by the prospect of losing the man she loved. All her life she had yearned to find someone to love and spend her life with; what a cruel twist of fate that having found him, he was about to die—at least according to the statistics—only three or four years into our relationship.

Before the pandemic, Leila and I went to meet a friend she had made on Facebook. Her name is Stephanie Bruneau, and her husband, Emile Bruneau, was a visiting scholar at the Annenberg School at the University of Pennsylvania, where he established the Peace and Conflict Neuroscience Lab. He was a neuroscientist and psychologist who tried to use those tools to work for peace, an effort that took him from South Africa to Colombia and many other conflict zones. In a strange way, we had parallel lives: they lived outside Philadelphia, as my family had; he had an extraordinary mother who lived through very difficult times; we worked in places that most people were trying to flee; and we were both diagnosed with GBM. He was diagnosed in 2018, and in September 2020 he died, at the age of forty-seven, leaving his wife, Stephanie, and their two children.

Instead of surrendering to this disease, however, he was determined to approach it with the kind of courage and mindfulness that many of us find difficult even when well. In January 2019, he brought together students and colleagues for a meeting at his home in Philadelphia, and that set the scene for a brief film about him, his work, and his illness. The handsome, lean young man, with bright blue eyes, a delicately chiseled face, and a salt-and-pepper beard, radiates vitality and goodness even on film. As he looked around at the people gathered there, he said that he appreciated the human experience of grieving for someone you care about, but at the same time, he wanted to share the perspective that he had on his illness. This was only a few weeks after he had been diagnosed with GBM. In his case, he didn't have some wild seizure but noticed that his computer monitor was getting darker and darker; no matter how much he turned on the brightness, it was still getting darker. Then he began getting headaches, and being a neuroscientist, he was "pretty sure that it was a tumor that was causing this, and it was a bad sign."

After a trip to urgent care, where a CT scan was performed, he was quickly sent to the hospital and admitted. Four days later, he was in surgery to remove a GBM tumor in his visual cortex. He was adept at reading medical research and saw the "bleak" survival curves. "I responded to this diagnosis in a way that I know I'm not supposed to respond. I'm supposed to go through the stages of grief . . . denial, anger, bereavement—these types of stages that are common for the human brain to go through," he said, as the film took us into his backyard. But he thought that there could be another way, and "one of them was to get this incredible sense of clarity." He realized that this was a blessing because he could focus on the things he wanted to achieve rather than the enormous losses he was facing. And he realized that one strategy for decreasing conflict is to appeal to empathy.

He talked about his death, but with remarkable equanimity. He began by explaining that everyone has their own time line for when they will die, an "uncomfortable reality," he called it. And no one knows when, or how, it will finally happen. He said that he was still on a time line, but the "probability curve is shifted. The maximum has decreased quite a bit," and he had more certainty on how he was going to die. He felt "fortunate" because he had some time to prepare his children for the loss of their father. The film then showed a picture of a beautiful young family, two children curled up with their parents, a picture of serenity and happiness. Providing his children with all the support that they would need to cope with the trauma of his death was another one of his missions for the time remaining.

He wondered why he responded so positively to this trauma. He said that his determination to do something positive in this world came from his mother. She had walked through "an incredible valley of darkness" but never made things difficult for him. Again, our experiences had some parallels—a shitty diagnosis and a mother who did so much for her children when she was burdened by many demands in a hard life. Just before his first brain surgery, he wrote Stephanie a letter, which she found on his computer: "I just had a thought: I learned in physics that our physical mass never actually touches another's—the outer electrons of each [atom] repel, giving us the illusion of touch. As a neuroscientist, I learned that our brains don't really see the world, they just interpret it. So, losing my body is not really a loss after all! What I am to you is really a reflection of your own mind. I am, and always was, there, in you."

We found out about Emile Bruneau when Leila met his widow on Facebook.

We reached out to Stephanie after he had died, and she kindly welcomed us. As we spoke, she offered us one important piece of advice. She said that what she most regretted about Emile's death was that they did not take time to grieve together when they still could, and she wished that they had done that. Having read about him, and seen the YouTube film made about him, I could see that his positive attitude, however bracing and impressive, may also have left little room for the profound grief that the two must have faced as a couple. They would be deprived of the simple pleasures of watching together as their children grew up and deepening the experience of their life together through the years. As Stephanie spoke, we could almost feel his presence among us, but the power of his absence and her loss was still greater. He was so young, and no matter how well-prepared he was, no matter how intentional his last years of life were, the loss for his wife and children is irreducible. Stephanie shared with us the importance of grieving these things.

Leila and I took this to heart, and together we began to grieve, not exactly over my death, of course, because that hasn't happened yet. I still believe I will not succumb to GBM, and moreover, I believe that boundless optimism is my greatest weapon in my own private war against this cerebral thief. No, thanks to Stephanie Bruneau, Leila and I began to grieve for the life together that we had *already* lost: our London home, the activities and the experiences we shared that will never be replicated, the places we can no longer go to, the ease of our existence that we once took for granted. I might have managed to do more, of course, as an almost able-bodied person. Maybe I could have returned to London, and we could have continued going to poetry readings or dining with friends. But thanks to COVID-19, that too became impossible for someone like me, who is immunocompromised. Another loss layered on top of the grief from my brain tumor.

And yet, there remains a special purity in simply being deeply linked. We have distilled our lives into the things that matter, and what matters is whatever kind of life we can manage—together. So yes, perhaps my illness is not a laughing matter. Except I still cannot ignore the many ways in which it is. And make the best I can out of a shitty deal.

"THEY BUILT LIBRARIES TO HONOR LOVED ONES, WOMEN FELLED BY BOMBINGS"

Coauthored by Fatima Faizi

New York Times

February 21, 2021

KABUL, Afghanistan—When his soon-to-be fiancée, Najiba Hussaini, was killed in a Taliban suicide bombing in Kabul, Hussain Rezai didn't know how to grieve for her.

"I had lost my love, but I wasn't allowed to mourn," said Mr. Rezai, a 33-year-old government employee. Though they had traveled to Daikundi Province to seek her parents' approval to marry, they weren't officially engaged, and he felt pressure to simply move on after her death.

It was July 2017 when a Taliban bomber detonated a vehicle packed with explosives, killing at least 24 people, including Ms. Hussaini, who was 28.

Thirteen months later, on the other side of the city, 40 students were killed when an Islamic State bomber detonated himself at a university entrance exam preparation center. Among those killed was Rahila Monji, 17, the youngest of nine siblings.

These women didn't know each other, but their lives were snuffed out by the same uncompromising violence that has killed thousands and left gaping holes in the lives of countless Afghans.

Yet Ms. Hussaini and Ms. Monji's loved ones were inspired to fulfill the same dream: to build public libraries memorializing the women they had lost.

Today, those libraries—one in Kabul, the capital, and the other in Daikundi Province—stand as symbols of the progress made toward gender equality and access to education in Afghanistan, where as many as 3.5 million girls are enrolled in school, according to a recent U.S. watchdog report, and where, as of 2018, one-third of the nation's teachers were women. . . .

"Najiba is not dead, she breathes with all the girls and boys who come to her library and study," Mr. Rezai said. . . .

"Now my sister saves the lives of hundreds of others," said Hamid Omer, Ms. Monji's brother. "Her soul is inside each of them."

CHAPTER 17

The Meaning of Life
(Is More Than Forty-Two)

One of the advantages of having a terminal illness is that it gives you a certain license to say things to people and ask things of people you wouldn't or couldn't ordinarily do. I now find openings to ask people what they think the meaning of life is. It comes up often in this way. I'll be on a long call with somebody and at the end they'll give me my opening: "Is there anything else I can do for you, Mr. Nordland?"

"No, not unless you could tell me the meaning of life," I'll say. Usually, people know that I have a terminal illness, so they take the question seriously. Answers have ranged from sad to profound, poignant to religious, trite to sometimes just downright funny. I asked a gravedigger at a cemetery (who was using a backhoe, not a shovel), and he replied ruefully, "'Life is a bitch and then you die,' as the saying goes."

I responded gamely, trying to lighten the moment. "I thought the saying was 'Life is a beach and then you die.'"

"That's just ridiculous," he said, laughing a little strangely. Oh well. My anger management therapist, John Tiedemann of New York City, had this answer: "Well, I don't know the meaning of life, but I do know the secret of finding happiness: be who you say you are."

I even asked my Alexa, expecting her to demur, but instead she quoted Eleanor Roosevelt: "Eleanor Roosevelt said that 'the purpose of life is to live it, to taste experience to the utmost, to reach out eagerly and without fear for newer and richer experience.'"

I suppose she did that indeed.

"To know that I have honored my ancestors," said a Hispanic day laborer wearing a big cross on a gold chain, whom I met on a footpath beside the Hudson River one Sunday morning last spring; we were both drenched from a heavy downpour, which I was enjoying immensely. He was on his way to church.

"How are you?" he asked.

"Well, other than terminal cancer, I'm doing just fine," I said— my standard reply to that common question.

"God bless you," he said. "I'll light a candle for you. What are you up to today?"

"Well, to be honest, I'm wandering around asking people about the meaning of life for a book I'm writing." In quite a few cases people have promptly answered, "Forty-two." This is a reference to Douglas Adams's *The Hitchhiker's Guide to the Galaxy*, in which the greatest supercomputer ever built comes up with forty-two as the answer to "life, the universe, and everything." But it turns out that the computer, comically, doesn't know what the question was.

One of the funniest replies I got to the question was from a woman in a call center in Texas, who immediately responded in a lovely, heavy Texan drawl: "Honey, you think if I knew the answer to that question, I'd be working in a call center for fifteen dollars an hour?" My assistant Taylor had a great off-the-cuff answer: "I'll get back to you on that." I'm still waiting for him to do so.

On one occasion I asked the nurse in my doctor's office what she thought the meaning of life was, and she challenged me to give my answer first. So I said, "I'm afraid I'm going to have to punt on that and just quote the writer Raymond Carver in his last poem in the book of poetry he wrote when he was dying of lung cancer, *A New Path to the Waterfall*. In this poem someone considers the question 'And did you get what you wanted from life?' The answer: 'I did.'

"'And what was it?'

"'To know that I am beloved on the earth.'"

And that's my answer too; now I do feel beloved on the earth. I now know how deeply beloved I am, by my children and family, by my friends, by a lot of people. I will die happy, knowing that. And that has given meaning to my life; without my tumor and its awful prognosis, I never would have learned that. So that was my answer. The nurse was a bit overwhelmed. She didn't expect that. Her own answer was a terse "Forty-two."

The writer Gloria Emerson, the first female war correspondent to cover Vietnam for the *New York Times* and the winner of the National Book Award for her stunning book on Vietnam, *Winners and Losers*, was both a mentor and a kind of second mother to me and my photographer friend Matthew Naythons. We both became especially close to her after our own mothers had died, mine of cervical cancer in 1994, at the age of sixty-four, Matthew's of a stroke in the 1980s. Gloria delivered the eulogy at my mother's funeral—she had befriended my mother in her later years (which Gloria mostly spent as a tireless advocate for Vietnam vets), seeing something special in her and endearing herself to us all as a result. Gloria even addressed my mother as "Mickey," her family nickname. "I have never seen anyone who was so loved," she said in her eulogy.

A few years earlier, my mother had contracted the now preventable and often curable disease cervical cancer, and was diagnosed at stage 4, giving her, the oncologist said, only a few months to live. Then, when one of her daughters or daughters-in-law became pregnant, my mother vowed she would live long enough to see a grandchild born. That set off a population explosion in our family; all of us had dreamed of reproducing the happy family of six we grew up in, happy despite all the adversity—this gave us added incentive. One of my sisters had six kids, another five, a brother five, and even I managed between wars to help make three—the fewest of us all. My mother kept her side of the bargain as long as she possibly could, and by the time she did finally die, nearly five years later, she had nineteen grandchildren. If she were alive now, she would get to meet all twenty-five of them. And more than ten great-grandchildren.

Susan Walker, the wife of a friend, once asked Gloria what she thought the meaning of life was; Gloria snapped at her with cynicism bordering on rage: "Oh Susan Walker, don't you know there is no meaning to life?" Perhaps not surprisingly, after Gloria came down with Parkinson's disease, losing her mobility and independence and in terrible pain, she committed suicide in 2004, at the age of seventy-five. Her funeral was held in a packed Friends Meeting House on Stuyvesant Square; many of us there were brokenhearted to lose her. If she could have seen the love and grief that filled that spacious hall, I like to think that she would never have been able to leave us all so abruptly, nor to think that a life like hers could ever be considered bereft of meaning.

I think that is a good thought exercise for anyone contemplating taking the "easy way out": imagine your own funeral, crowded with broken hearts.

"IS THE LIGHT AT THE END OF THIS TUNNEL THE BEAM OF AN ONCOMING TRAIN?"

New York Times
April 26, 2020

Having been a war correspondent much of my life, I can't shake the feeling that the war against the coronavirus is a lot like the real thing.

Normally, I would avoid using a war metaphor for a medical disaster, if only because it has been so loosely applied by so many politicians doomed to failure: Consider Lyndon Johnson's war on poverty, Nixon's war on cancer and his war on drugs, which Ronald Reagan escalated, making it an unending "war" to this day.

But the coronavirus war is something new, if only in the terrible toll it has taken in lives and the way it has altered the lives of the rest of us.

Like so many others in New York, to which I retreated months ago for surgery and a long recuperation, I now suddenly find myself in quarantine to be sure I don't acquire the coronavirus. Not since the siege of Sarajevo three decades ago have I been forcibly cooped up in the same building for weeks, afraid to step outside for fear of some life-changing—or life-ending—encounter.

CHAPTER 18

Solitary Confinement

The months after my surgery and chemo at the end of 2019 were consumed by trips to my oncologist, physical therapist, occupational therapist, psychotherapist, and hand therapist. I had brain scans every few months, which I approached with almost giddy optimism, certain that once more I would beat the odds and show this terrible disease that it may have met its match. Leila had to return to London for work for a spell, so as not to overstay her visa and to earn a living. Our times apart were difficult for both of us. But we soldiered on, and this very constrained life of mine was bolstered by my connection with her, my children, my large family, and friends. I was living my Second Life with gratitude and hope. Yes, I was impaired. Still am, really, but I was alive, and every day that I moved further from my seizures and surgery was a day to celebrate.

I will not belabor my impulsive decision to hop on a bicycle and go for a ride in Midtown Manhattan. It was January 2020, the holidays had been especially festive, and now that I was pretty much on my own, I felt the need to be more mobile. I hopped on a normal bicycle, which, given my post-operative problems with stability and proprioception (just standing on the wood floors of my apartment poses challenges), was a catastrophically bad idea. I had also underestimated the aggressiveness of New York City cyclists—the bike messengers and the people who deliver meals and groceries and the simple commuters, many of whom are intense, often reckless riders. And yet I reasoned that I was also an experienced bicyclist, having ridden the three thousand miles across the United States in my late teens. But nothing prepared me for encountering the electric bike, going the wrong way in the bike lane, against the arrows, at a very high speed—and heading right for me. The rider sideswiped me while traveling probably thirty miles per hour. I flew off the bike, landing hard, breaking . . . something. Before the tumor I would probably have managed to maneuver out of the biker's way, but as I've been reminded time and again, I am no longer physically the person I used to be. The biker didn't even pause to see how I was, let alone stop to render assistance.

The emergency room doctor initially thought that I had suffered a broken rib, the clinical lesson being that when you look for something hard enough, you tend to find it. Since they were looking for a broken rib, that's what they found. The pain was intense, which, I was told, was normal. Broken ribs typically heal on their own, so there was not much to be done except endure the pain as best as I could. What they did not see on the x-ray—I suppose because they were not looking for it—was that my back was also broken. My spine was fractured in three places, further complicated by severe stenosis of the lumbar vertebrae, which pressed against my nerves and caused pain to emanate around my hips and down my legs. When I complained about excruciating pain, I was told that it was probably just arthritis.

When I next saw Dr. Fine—who had cautioned me against bicycling—I immediately said, "Don't bother telling me 'I told you so,' Doc, 'cause I've already done that for you."

One of the (few) great things about my fatal brain tumor is that unlike many cancers—lung or mouth or especially pancreatic— it hasn't been painful. As I've mentioned, I've been afflicted with chemo brain, but a certain vagueness and forgetfulness, as inconvenient as that is, was nothing compared to the consuming and chronic pain that I experienced after my accident. Pain took over my entire life. I was barely able to walk. I was terribly depressed, waking up from a blissful night's sleep pleased to be alive but wondering, what next now? I feared falling into the possibly bottomless abyss of depression. What a painful irony that a brain tumor had never led me to this dark place, but a bike collision did.

The doctors would not give me opioids out of fear that I would get addicted. Dr. Fine recalled that early on, I had said to my doctor, "Whatever you do, don't give me opioids because I'm a highly addictive personality." Plus their side effects could interfere with both chemotherapy and the anti-seizure meds I was on. Finally, my posse of doctors—brain surgeon, head oncologist, chief neurologist, palliative care specialist, rheumatologist, and primary care physician—conferred and debated whether I could have Percocet occasionally to cope with the breakthrough pain. I met with my rheumatologist, Dr. Yuan, and begged for Percocet, hoping that she might become my advocate with my other doctors. This could not possibly be arthritis.

Late one night I was so desperate that I contemplated going out on Times Square to try to score Percocet from a drug dealer; fortunately my partner, Leila, prevented me from taking that foolish step. At my lowest point, I was reduced to using a walker.

I had an MRI, and the scan revealed that my spine was fractured in three places; there was also stenosis of several vertebrae, further exacerbating the pain. At last, we knew its cause, and that presented the possibility of spinal surgery to end it. But when pain is so intense, when the simple act of breathing or walking to the kitchen to make coffee is agonizing, the vague sense that relief may come with surgery in the future is utterly meaningless. I was in a kind of solitary confinement within my body, and I had to find ways to cope.

Once more the hospital became my lifeline, this time through its department of integrative health and well-being. The department studied and offered mindfulness and meditation-based stress reduction (MMBSR), acupuncture, therapeutic massage, and other options once considered the woo-woo domain of counterculture fringe types. Even now, many people do not associate these practices with cutting-edge modern medicine. Earlier in life I would have derided them as hippy-dippy nonsense. But over the years, gold-standard medical research has proved their effectiveness and persuaded insurance companies to pay for them. I relied on all the offerings, especially the mindfulness meditation—breathing and listening to tapes and instruction—while I waited for surgery. Still, it wasn't sufficient to cope with the consuming torment. Acupuncture sometimes gave me relief for a few hours—about as much as one Percocet does. I was shocked when the acupuncturist put needles in my right earlobe to address the pain in my left hip joint. When he did, I felt, or thought I felt, something like a low-level electric current pass between my ear and the pain point in my hip. I never would have believed this was possible if I hadn't experienced it myself—and each session at least gave me fleeting relief.

I still managed to keep going, did the physical therapy exercises assigned to me first thing in the morning, and then went straight out for a half-mile walk, feeling as if I were learning how to walk again. The half mile soon became a full mile from time to time, and every day became easier. I walked more like someone who knew how to do it. I also noticed that after a mile the pain disappeared. It got to the point that I'd be able to tell when I had walked a mile simply because suddenly the pain would stop. I would check my watch or my phone and see, indeed, that I had just gone a mile; it felt hopeful. I was getting ready for my back surgery when, in yet another ill-conceived but energetic effort, I decided to paint and sand some furniture. I fell, cracked my head open, and ended up in the hospital once more. Back surgery yet again postponed. My physical therapist warned me to stop using the walker, or my walking muscles would atrophy and I'd be using it for life. Best advice I ever got. I threw the accursed thing away and never went back to it.

So I muddled through. I was able to visit friends or receive them at my apartment or go out and have dinner, enjoy the pleasures of New York. I spent a lot of time in the Rose Reading Room of the New York Public Library, writing and reading.

Around that time, I decided to take a six-month Introduction to Judaism course offered online by a Brooklyn synagogue. My studies, which I could do from the apartment by Zoom, largely consisted of analyzing and discussing the weekly Torah portion—the *parsha*. I learned that if you read each week's *parsha*, you will have completed the entire Torah, or five books of Moses, by the end of a year. I began to feel that I had found the spiritual home I had long yearned for.

The rabbi who taught my course told a story that struck me as I faced mortality within my confined physical circumstances: Some rich men were discussing how they might carry their wealth with them on a long journey. What form should it take? They think gold bars will be too heavy. Then their rabbi tells them, "You don't have to worry about how heavy it is. Your riches have no weight at all. They are the knowledge you have in your head, and you will carry that always. Your knowledge is your most valuable possession of all."

In the course of my studies, I gained respect for the willingness I found among Jewish people to question God, and not blindly take the *mitzvot*—or commandments—as God's incontrovertible law. I learned of their long tradition of this questioning, which began with Moses and Abraham, through to Job, who all argued with God. I had found the place for me.

I worried—especially after I decided to convert—that as a life-long atheist I might be asked "Do you believe in God?" but this in fact never came up. As Bernard-Henri Lévy says in *The Genius of Judaism*, "No Jew is required to believe in God." The Jews use reason, intellect, and questioning to make sense of the world, which appealed to me deeply.

But then came March 2020, and the coronavirus consumed New York. Going outside was dangerous, visiting anywhere was danger-ous, the Rose Room at the New York Public Library was closed for a long time, as was the whole New York Public Library. Any visitors to my apartment had to go through the rigmarole of putting on ICU-level PPE to enter, so they finally stopped coming. And even if they did want to, I was so immunocompromised and the virus was so infectious, it was impossible to keep my anxiety—and es-pecially Leila's anxiety on my behalf—at bay. I tried to arrange to meet people in Central Park for socially distanced walks and talks, but more people agreed to that than actually did it. Not everyone enjoys going on walks in the park, and my back injury made those rambles an ordeal.

I felt utterly alone. I would get in touch with friends and family on FaceTime or email. I would try to make my appointments but often forgot when they were supposed to take place. My hair got wild, and I became disoriented, with all my reliable points of refer-ence gone. The limited life I had constructed for myself unraveled. Leila, my kids, my friends were all afraid for me because I was on my own, and no one was there to look after me. What if I fell? What if I had a terrible seizure? During the first two months especially, no one could figure out a way to keep me safe. Leila remembers being on FaceTime with me for hours, just watching to see how I was do-ing. Chemo and the tumor destroyed my capacity to be fully aware of what was going on much of the time. Add to that the catastrophic isolation of lockdown in the city, and I found myself experiencing what solitary confinement must be like. Because I was in solitary confinement. And I felt as if I was indeed slowly going mad.

When I was reporting from the war in Iraq, I became interested in investigating the way the United States treated and engaged in human rights abuses of prisoners. The prison in Abu Ghraib, the renditions in Guantánamo Bay, and the massive garden-variety depravity visited on those taken into custody were a major preoccupation for me. One of the special favorite forms of torture, infamously approved by American leaders, was solitary confinement, which takes a severe toll.

As I was thinking about the implications of solitary confinement, I read a seminal study of rhesus monkeys written by Harry Harlow at the University of Wisconsin in the 1950s. He found that "twelve months of isolation almost obliterated the animals socially." The monkeys often resorted to head banging and other forms of self-harm, which also happen frequently to people in solitary confinement. Terry Anderson, the Associated Press reporter in Beirut who was held as a hostage for almost seven years, was one of many such hostages who reported that his mind seemed to disintegrate through lack of stimulation; he forgot books he had read, poems he had memorized, until, finally, he wrote, "There's nothing there, just a formless, gray-black misery. My mind's gone dead."

Muscles atrophy steadily with disuse, losing as much as 50 percent of their mass in a month's time with no movement at all, 25 percent of their mass in a month in a room with limited mobility or when the person is shackled or otherwise restrained. That sort of loss of muscle mass, occurring through a process known medically as cachexia, or wasting disease, makes standing and even sitting difficult. One of the first signs that atrophy has reached catastrophic levels is when the act of sitting up, normally the body's most comfortable and least challenging position, results in severe pain across the buttocks, both in assuming the position and in trying to hold it. Standing for more than a few moments becomes extremely difficult and walking impossible. Rehabilitation requires slow rebuilding of the muscle mass, a process that can take many months, even after a relatively short period of confinement.

In many cases of confinement, but particularly for hostages, light is severely restricted, and eyesight so adapts to the darkness that sudden exposure to light can be extremely painful. In severe cases, this can lead to photokeratitis, a condition akin to what happens to an arc welder without eye protection, or in cases of snow blindness at high altitudes. Photokeratitis is characterized by intense pain, uncontrollable tearing from both eyes, and constricted pupils; it may persist for hours or for days. In particularly bad cases, it results in blepharospasm, the involuntary closure of the eyelids for long periods, followed by severe twitching of the eyelids, a condition that can prove incurable.

I thought about Iraq and my interest in solitary confinement during 2020, when I found myself facing a kind of solitary confinement in the middle of New York City that I had never imagined possible. And through other people's reactions to me, I could see myself psychologically disintegrating.

I cannot remember all the details about how Leila took the enormous risk of air travel at the height of the coronavirus pandemic, when New York City was for a time its epicenter in America, and came to stay with me. But Leila later reminded me of what I missed. It must have been in the summer of 2020. She arrived in New York and came immediately to my apartment. I still remember the look of shock on her face. I must have appeared quite deranged, my hair long, a haunted expression on my face. My apartment was a disaster.

It seemed to her—and to me, when I summoned up the courage to look in the mirror—that I had gone feral.

It had become impossible for me to maintain order in my surroundings, and of course I couldn't permit a cleaning person inside because of the great risk that it posed for infection, since such working people used mass transportation. I had a couple score of tropical fish I had put in the drip trays of the jungle of plants I was cultivating in my apartment; then I got a pair of parakeets for company and let them out on walkabouts—they always returned to their cage because that's where their food and water was. But they carried out a genocide on the fishes, which all disappeared overnight, no doubt down those skinny parakeet necks. I myself started to smell bad, partly for lack of bathing due to my fear of falling in the bathtub. My apartment had that dangerous shower-over-tub arrangement, so I would allow myself to bathe only when someone responsible was present. It is a true friend who can tell you that you smell bad, as my old friend Larry did around that time. One day "Keet One" (I never gave them names other than Keet One and Two) went on her usual walkabout and pecked at the bait in a spring-loaded mousetrap, which broke her neck. I promptly defenestrated her body, and I swear I heard, or thought I heard, a lady shriek in the street twelve floors below. Then Keet 2 went on a forlorn walkabout looking for his mate and never returned to his cage. A housekeeper (I had given in and hired one) and I searched everywhere for the bird but never found a trace. Our best guess was that it had followed its mate out an open window—perishing because its clipped wings prevented flying.

Before the pandemic, I was happy. I was sustained by the love that surrounded me. But in the solitary confinement of the pandemic, often with pain as my only companion, I felt as if Terry Anderson's observation about his ordeal was my own: "There's nothing there, just a formless, gray-black misery. My mind's gone dead."

But Leila was now with me. And a year after the pandemic began, I was vaccinated against COVID in a high school gym in Queens. When I got my injection, it brought tears of joy to my eyes. And as the aftereffects of chemo wore off, I found I could write and think clearly once more. And I felt like Leila and I still had a future, however difficult it might be.

"THE KABUL BUREAU'S ACCIDENTAL GARDENER"
New York Times
May 24, 2019

KABUL, Afghanistan . . .

Gardens are one of Kabul's secret pleasures. The city is on a high desert plateau, but behind all those blast walls and shabby modern buildings, many Kabul homes hide luscious blooms: fruit trees and plants that flower for months on end. With 300 days of sunshine a year, things grow with gusto so long as there is water, and our original bureau had a deep well to draw on. A little greenhouse sheltered plants that could not survive the short but harsh winter. . . .

The garden is not often the first thing on our minds, as we cover Afghanistan's long war. I didn't notice what was going on until one day last year I looked out the window in front of my desk on the second floor and saw the purple floral spike of a hollyhock at eye level, a good 12 feet above the flower beds. It would grow another three feet before succumbing to gravity. There were sunflowers, too, that were nearly as tall. Rampant vines colonized the compound walls, disguising some of the ugliness of the inevitable fortifications. . . .

The garden is so splendid we have added a hammock—rarely used, but beckoning.

CHAPTER 19

My Last War

To have been a foreign correspondent who covered Afghanistan on and off for nearly forty years, including the past nine years straight, then to be sidelined by a brain tumor during the painfully historic moment when the Taliban came back to power in August 2021, during a disastrous exit by the United States, was to feel an incomparable level of frustration and despair. I knew this story. I had the contacts. I had been in regular touch with Zabihullah Mujahid, the Taliban spokesman and the head of their media department. In the past, with the help of our interpreters, we would play out all the potential scenarios. I knew that when a government was as corrupt as the one supported by the United States, it was inevitable that the Taliban would eventually triumph and return.

Which is just what happened. I had even asked the Taliban spokesman through an interpreter whether it would be safe for me to remain in Kabul, and he assured me it would be. Whatever else the Taliban spokesman was, I believed, and had ample evidence to support the belief, that he was a man of his word. Once, years earlier, the American official in charge of what they called strategic communications asked me what the Taliban were doing better than the Americans in interacting with the American media. At the time this was an American flag officer named Admiral Greg Smith. I earned

his probably undying enmity by suggesting that he invite Zabihullah Mujahid, the Taliban spokesman, to a handling-the-media sem-
inar with the American military, which I said I would be happy to
arrange—a proposal that was only slightly tongue in cheek.

"Seriously," he said, "what do they do that we don't?"

"Well, for starters, their default position is to tell the truth. If
you ask them about something and they can't answer honestly, they
say so; if they promise to investigate and get back to us, they do,
in hours, not after months of fruitless investigation. And they are
always far quicker than you guys at responding to us."

"That's because they don't have to worry about getting the truth,
and we do," the admiral said.

"You do?" I said. "I'd say on that score you're about tied." I
immediately recalled the time I was working on a story about the
problematic US efforts to rebuild the Afghan military. There was an
interview I had with the Afghan general in charge of the helicopter
wing, which was in the process of getting scores of new helicopters
designed by the Americans for the Afghan Air Force. As a horrified
American public affairs officer, a colonel, listened aghast and tried
in vain to get the Afghan general to shut up, the general proceeded
to ridicule the new helicopter, saying it was unable to reach an alti-
tude high enough to clear the mountains ringing Kabul, where they
were to be based. It was also poorly armed and inadequately armored.
They could not even stay aloft in much of the country, due to the
thinner air at high elevations.

But instead of being there, in the midst of the chaos and yet another transformation of that country, I was in New York, reading everything that I could. I tried to keep up by talking with a few of my
colleagues, especially Alissa Rubin. She was part of the *Times* team
that had been mobilized to evacuate and resettle our Afghan staff and
their families, 281 people who were certain to be targets of the new
government. All the people who had made our lives possible there—

the fixers and drivers, the cooks and the translators, the bodyguards and security detail—were facing mortal danger for the simple reason that they had worked for us, or were related to someone who had. As I watched the chaotic scenes at the airport, I thought of how many times I had flown in and out of it, I thought of the stories I did, the people I knew, and my conviction that what was unfolding now before me had been inevitable, as many of my stories here have demonstrated. Not to be a part of it now seemed inconceivable.

And yet I had moved into a different theater of war, one with negligible international implications but cataclysmic personal ones. I learned over the years that if there was a single golden rule for reporting from a conflict zone, it was this: you need an exit plan because you must live to tell the story. One always needs some strategy for removing oneself as quickly and safely as possible, should things get out of control—which they so often do. If it gets too dangerous, how is one to get out? This golden rule, it turns out, is true both geopolitically and personally. As I watched the mess at the Kabul airport, I could see that the United States clearly did not have anything resembling a coherent exit plan—much less any indication that they had weighed the risks in a thoughtful way. In the war in which I find myself now, a battle for my life, the exit plan is more difficult to configure. What does it look like to escape from GBM-4?

In every story we do in a war zone, there's a calculation at the base of it, the risk versus the reward. I'm accustomed to calculating survival odds. Just making it alive to the publication of this book will beat the odds of 6 or 7 percent. From diagnosis to death at my age, the median life expectancy for GBM was fifteen months, meaning the bottom date on my tombstone should have been roughly November 5, 2020—age seventy-one. I am writing this in 2023—which means, as my old war correspondent buddy George de Lama put it, I am now, and have been for almost two years, "playing with the house's money."

I suppose that there are objective reasons for why my risk ratio has turned out to be a lot better than the official prognostication. I'm getting world-class care in a world-class hospital and I'm physically healthy. I've had many clear brain scans, with no sign of return or spread of the tumor. But the cold reality is that I have no idea if, when you are reading this, you will be able to google my obituary or sign up to see me at your local bookstore. I am prepared. If there was ever a life designed to teach one how to face death, mine was it.

Sometimes my exit plan becomes a thought experiment. I wonder if I can just buy some more time, "play for the come," as we say in poker, where I can keep the worst of the catastrophe at bay, muddling through with my therapy sessions and my rather limited life, until a brand-new, miraculous treatment for GBM is discovered. A treatment that will completely eradicate errant cancer cells and maybe energize the brain's plasticity so as to repair whatever region had been violated. As I daydream about this exit plan, I imagine seeing these few years of frailty and illness as an intermezzo in my rich and engaged life.

But I am a realist, aware that this may well not happen. No matter how many billions have been spent on the cancer moonshot in Beau Biden's memory, who knows how much will be allocated for GBM, and even then, the length of time it takes from promising treatment to the market is, quite literally for many of us, a lifetime.

So that means that an essential part of my exit plan is being realistic in calculating my losses. I may well not see any of my children marry, or cradle a grandchild in my arms. I may well never return to Kabul or London or Rome, perhaps the only city on earth I can navigate by memory without GPS, so intimately do I know it. In many ways it made me the person I am—the first place where I covered a country I didn't know in a language I couldn't then speak, the first where I managed a foreign bureau. I may never return to any of the places where I've worked and loved. I will cover no more foreign wars, even as new ones burst onto the scene. I have lost some friends, but I have reconciled with others. I may not grow old with Leila, sit companionably with her in some lovely place we can call our own as we both read or write, noticing her hair turning silver as mine goes from almost blond to white. I may not visit the magical Adirondacks camp of my dearest friend Alissa again, or have another sailing or safari adventure with Matthew, trading quips: "Food is fuel," "One word is worth a thousand pictures, even the definite article," "Plenty of time to sleep when you die." The last is a line I've bored so many people with that I became convinced it was my own—until I learned that both Ben Franklin and William Shakespeare beat me to it by hundreds of years.

Ah, the places I've gone, the people I've seen (to honor Dr. Seuss for a moment). The French neuroscientist David Servan-Schreiber, who also was stricken with glioblastoma, put it like this: "The approach of death can sometimes lead to a kind of liberation. Wouldn't it be far worse to have no reason to be sad at that moment of parting? And the finality of that moment forces us to recognize the profoundness of our love." Servan-Schreiber is my GBM hero: He survived a couple decades with the disease, long enough to write three terrific books. He was so widely loved and admired, it seemed that his funeral was attended by the whole of France.

Expressions of love sometimes come from unexpected quarters. I was a Nieman fellow at Harvard in 1988–89, and a friend of mine from that time, Mike Connor, wrote to me after he heard about my illness, responding to a missive I had earlier fired off to him.

Dear Rod,

It was the night of the first or maybe second time the Niemans gathered that late summer of '88 at Harvard. We had all just been introduced. You announced to the group that

The Ramones would take the stage downtown that night. Any
takers? Peter Richmond and I said heck yeah.

We watched from the wings for a while; soon a mosh pit
formed. As I remember it, you slipped off your leather jacket
and headed straight into the action. You emerged, eventually,
a bit bloodied—and buoyant. I stayed in the wings. I barely
knew you but knew I was witnessing a different kind of spirit:
Dauntless, willing to throw yourself literally into the heart of
experience to know it and tell it first-hand.

Through the years, I witnessed from afar with deepening
admiration as you did just that: Brought passion and daring
to your work, leaping into the heart of hotspots to know it and
tell it.

And now, facing all you're facing (25 docs and seven
therapists?) this same spirit prevails. Bloodied, but buoyant.
Undaunted. A 65,000-word book? It is epic life energy.

If I do get to NYC I would love to see you and drop off a
book (no flowers) if you're up to it at the time.

Meanwhile, I wish you no ceasing from adventure.

> *Your long-out-of-touch classmate,*
> *Mike*

Could there be a more blessed wish than one that involves "no
ceasing from adventure"? I have reread Mike's letter often; if it had
been on paper it would be soft and crumpled by now, not just for
the rekindling of a long-forgotten memory, but for the love and respect with which it was written. He *saw* me then, and sees me now,
so many decades hence.

The recognition of love, indeed, is a fundamental component of
my exit plan. I sometimes feel that eventuality of my death creeping
closer, just because I'm so far past the terrifyingly short median life
expectancy from a GBM-4 diagnosis. Yes, I continue to get clear

scans showing no glioblastoma progression, no new cancer, no new tumors or spread. My seizures are under control. My balance is terrible, but that is manageable. I can now button my shirts and put my pants on the right way around. My left hand has even revived a bit. Thanks to that neuroplasticity of the brain, I am teaching it to control the left hand visually, rather than by sensation; thus I can button shirts and tie shoelaces on my own again. Two-handed touch typing is a bigger challenge, but I am slowly learning to do it again, only at thirty words per minute now, but as my hand therapist Emily Altman pointed out, that is six times faster than my baseline when they tested me post-surgery. If I continue to progress like that, I'll be typing at a respectable speed in another year.

When I feel the cold breath of mortality down my neck, I counter it with a sense of gratitude. And I can still write a hundred words per minute—in longhand, which is how most of this book was written (then dictated to someone or to a speech-transcribing program). I still make my bed every morning, as I always have—even when there were helpers to do it for me. (I've always done that even in hotels and even, when I physically could, in hospitals, motivated by a superstition that the day I don't make my own bed will be the day I die.)

"How does your book end?" Jake asked innocently after I told him I'd finished the first rough draft. "I guess with my death," I almost said, but held my tongue. "Don't all lives, in war or peace, end with death? Isn't that the way we all end?" But in fact, before my own ending, this book must end with an expression of love toward everyone in my life. I have been blessed with a remarkably enormous and loving family, five brothers and sisters (my sister Cindy tragically and unexpectedly died last year, indirectly saving my life in the process; a long story to be elsewhere told). And I am further blessed with a vast and wonderful extended family, twenty-plus marvelous nieces and nephews, and, most recently, a baker's dozen or so of lovely little great-nieces and great-nephews. Above all, I've been blessed with an enduring and indestructible love with my six-foot-tall poet and partner, Leila, fierce and strong and brilliant, creative and brave and beautiful, who has been by my side since the very beginning of this journey and for every single step of the way since and who will be there to help make our ending—if there is to be one, which I still refuse to accept—as beautiful as our beginning, with our improbable love triumphant throughout.

And too my beloved children, Lorine, Johanna, and Jake, who came back to me when I needed them most and helped dispel the darkness, and many deeply caring friends, to whom I feel overwhelmingly grateful. They helped me know, as Raymond Carver did, that I can call myself beloved upon this earth, come what may. In the meantime, I plan to keep making my bed every morning, and if I do have to die—I have yet to accept that as a given—know that I will die a happy man.

I am still waiting for the monsoon. It will color my actions as I wait—as we all wait. The tumor has changed my life for the better; it has become my teacher. If I survive it, so much the better. Even if I don't, that much will always be true, even unto the end of days.

PHOTO GALLERY

All photographs
copyright © Matthew Naythons
unless otherwise noted

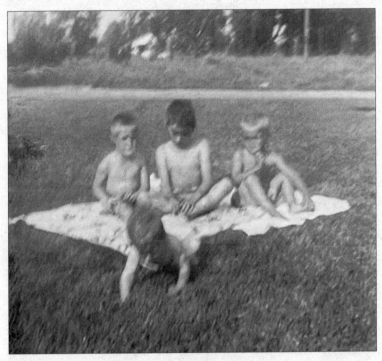

"The happy memories are in black and white." Rod Nordland (*center*) with siblings Gary, Craig, and Cindy, 1955. *Courtesy of the author*

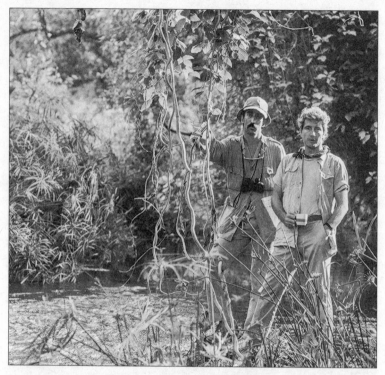

"What we lacked in adult supervision, we made up for in adventure." Victoria Falls National Park, Zimbabwe, 1984, after a morning jog along the Zambezi River amid a pride of lions, with photographer Matthew Naythons (*left*). © *Matthew Naythons Photographic Archive, Briscoe Center for American History, University of Texas at Austin*

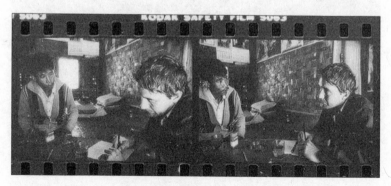

"Let them take us alive, please." Rebel territory, Burma, 1981, interviewing a Shan State Army officer. © *Matthew Naythons Photographic Archive, Briscoe Center for American History, University of Texas at Austin*

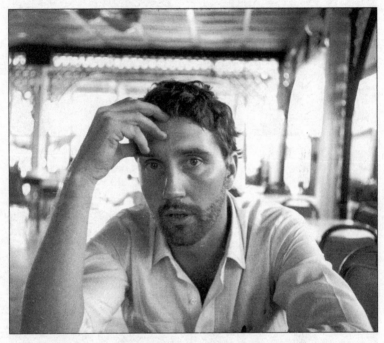
"The first time I saw a dead person, I saw a hundred of them." Thailand, 1979, at a refugee camp on the Thai-Cambodian border.

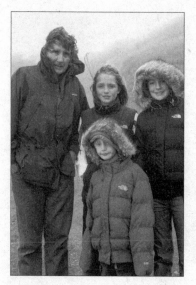

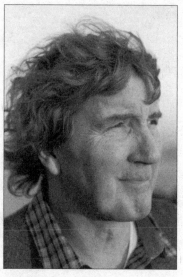

Family trip to San Francisco, 2006, with children Johanna, Lorine, and Jake.

"Millions of air miles." California, en route from Hong Kong to London, 2013.

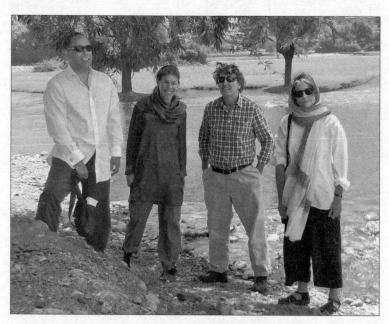

Afghanistan, with the *New York Times* team, 2013. *Left to right:* Dean Baquet, Alissa Rubin, Rod, Jill Abramson. *Courtesy of the author*

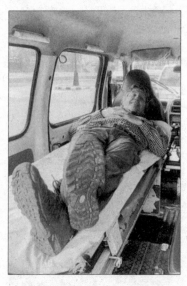

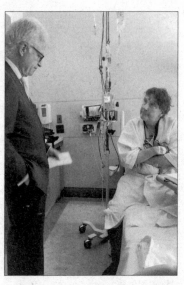

In the ambulance in New Delhi, July 2019, post-seizure. *Courtesy of the author*

"It's terminal. It's incurable. It will eventually kill you." With neurosurgeon Dr. Phil Stieg, New York-Presbyterian Hospital's Weill Cornell Medical Center.

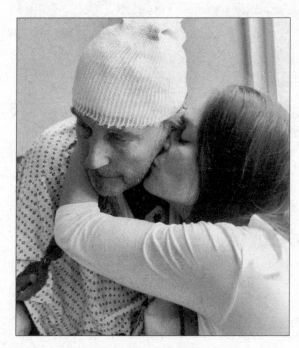

With Leila, after brain surgery to remove my tumor, July 2019.

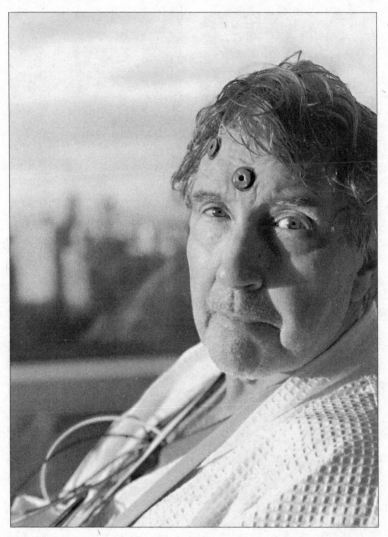

"I can call myself beloved upon this earth."

Acknowledgments

First of all I would like to thank the many medical personnel, doctors, nurses, and therapists who kept me alive and fully functional long enough to write this book—far longer than the median life expectancy upon diagnosis with glioblastoma multiforme stage 4, which is fifteen months. My diagnosis was forty-six months ago as I write, about the time it took me to complete this book.

I was blessed to get my care in New York City, which is so rich in world-class hospitals, including Weill Cornell Medical Center of the NewYork-Presbyterian Hospital, where I had my initial brain surgery, chemotherapy, and radiotherapy. Thank you to Philip Stieg, PhD, MD; Howard Fine, MD; Dana Leifer, MD; Silvia Formenti, MD; Jonathan Knisely, MD; Susan Pannullo, MD; Steven Karceski, MD; Robert Fakheri, MD, FACP; Lauren Costello, NP; Kris Hopkins, NP; Nicole Wenz, NP; Ivette Rivera; Dina Santamaria, RMA, RPT; and Leak Shalawn, LCSW.

When I broke my back in a post-onset bicycle accident, the injury was discovered by Weijia Yuan, MD, at the Hospital for Special Surgery, and fixed by Roger Hartl, MD, at Weill Cornell. Also at the Hospital for Special Surgery, my brilliant hand therapist, Emily Altman, DPT, helped me relearn how to tie my shoelaces and button my shirts; she taught me how to use my insensate left hand again. At Lenox Hill Hospital, John Boockvar, MD; Amy McKeown, NP-C;

Olivia Albers, FNP-BC; and their team were warm, compassionate, and generous with their time and advice.

Since my left hand was disabled by my brain tumor, I can only touch-type one-handed, which is painfully slow. So most of this book was written in longhand with my right hand, then dictated, and mostly transcribed, especially by my assistants Cassie Sheedy and Taylor Herrera. I owe them a huge debt of gratitude for their patience, endurance, and resourcefulness in this long and often tiresome work.

My literary agent, Suzanne Gluck of William Morris Endeavor, was a driving force in conceptualizing this book. The freelance editor and author Marianne Szegedy-Maszak did a wonderful job of helping me organize my material. My editor at HarperCollins, Peter Hubbard, VP and publisher, and leader of the Mariner imprint, has been pure joy to work with.

I am often asked by people, with more money than I to spare, where best to direct their charitable donations. I can't recommend any cancer charity more highly than CancerCare in New York, where William Goeren, LCSW; Sarah Kelly, LCSW; and Sheila Zablow gave always free advice that was insightful, wise, and practical. When it comes to glioblastoma, I would root for the Glioblastoma Foundation, where I received terrific advice for dealing with this horrible disease and helpful suggestions for this book.

Thanks also to Nicholas Parsons; Sally Silvers; Gregory Garritano, CPA; Katherine Gallusser; Gabriela Höhn, PhD; Evan Bracconeri, DPT; John Tiedemann; Sherry Zauderer; Andrea Jacobson; Celeste Meneses; Kwaku Gyamfi; Agnes Boateng; Leela Sookram; Deidre Baker; and the couples therapist Meigs Ross, LCSW, whose wisdom is beyond compare. Early on she gave Leila and me the best piece of advice ever: "Remember there are

now three parties in your relationship: Rod, Leila, and GBM"—
so true.

I am blessed with many dear friends and colleagues, who have
so often been there for me: Laurence and Carole Moskowitz, Alissa
Johannsen Rubin, Gary Knight, Jim Wiggins and Chris Fleming,
George and Carrie Holt de Lama, Robert Frump, Joseph Gold-
stein, Spencer Reiss, William McCarren, Tom Mathews, Betsy
Krebs and Sheldon Stein, Sam Clark and Susie Gannon, Mike
Connor, Josh Berger, Matthew Naythons, Duncan Wilson, David
Zucchino, Eugene Roberts Jr., Jasmine Cooray, Rowyda Amin,
Cass Bonner, Jayne Harvey, Severino Panzetta, and Barbara and
Michael Segal.

I have been further blessed with a generous and kind employer,
the *New York Times*, where so many people went above and beyond
the imaginable in supporting me. I could easily list hundreds of
Times folk but have space here to single out only a few: A. G. Sulz-
berger, Dean Baquet, Joseph Kahn, Marc Lacey, Michael Slack-
man, Douglas Schorzman, Grace Wong, Juanita Powell-Brunson,
Anthony Perry, Andria Greeney, Olaf Wilson, and Charlie
O'Malley. In India, thank you to Sunny Kumar Kangotra, and to
my *Times* colleagues Shalini Venugopal Bhagat, Suhasini Raj, Jeffrey Gettleman, and Jagmohan Bhakuni.

My three wonderful children, Lorine, Johanna, and Jake, have
given me more love and happiness than I ever expected possible.
My brothers and sisters, and in-laws, Darlene and Eutimeo Bruno,
Darrell Nordland, Craig and Lisa Nordland, Gary and Susan Nordland, and my late, much-missed sister Cynthia Bruno all gave me
tremendous support early in my illness. They also gave me more
than twenty nieces and nephews, not counting great-nieces and
great-nephews. Among them I would like to mention my nephew
Billy Bruno, MD, at Columbia and his wife, Kathryn Tringale,

MD, at Memorial Sloan Kettering, who were generous with advice and support, and my nephew William Bruno and his wife, Lauren, two of the best people I know.

Last and foremost I want to thank my devoted and loving partner, Leila Segal, who has done more than anyone to keep me alive. I am looking forward to the days to come with her, however many or few they may be.

Credits